THE NEUROPHYSIOLOGIC BASIS
OF PATIENT TREATMENT

VOLUME III   PERIPHERAL COMPONENTS OF MOTOR CONTROL

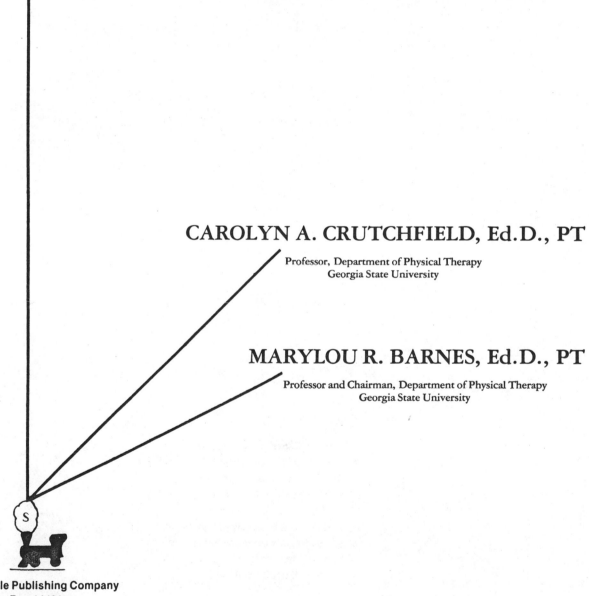

CAROLYN A. CRUTCHFIELD, Ed.D., PT

Professor, Department of Physical Therapy
Georgia State University

MARYLOU R. BARNES, Ed.D., PT

Professor and Chairman, Department of Physical Therapy
Georgia State University

Stokesville Publishing Company
Box 14401
Atlanta, GA 30324

TABLE OF CONTENTS

INTRODUCTION AND INSTRUCTIONS

INTRODUCTION AND INSTRUCTIONS

In this volume we have attempted to present relevant applied neurophysiology of the peripheral nervous system. You should not infer from such an approach that the peripheral system is meant to stand in isolation from the knowledge and application of higher level functions. The term motor control carries with it the connotation of higher level functioning in which supraspinal centers decide the fate of movement outcomes. While such a view is true in a large sense, there are many effects and modifications of motor behavior made by peripheral and spinal interactions. Movement results, however, from the integration of reflexes, automatic or pre-programmed circuits and voluntary pathways. Movement requires both peripheral and supraspinal circuits.

We believe that to understand the effects of sensory manipulation, it is necessary to have some knowledge of the motor systems upon which such sensory input impacts. For this reason Section I has been included in this text. The study of sensory function begins in Section II. The anatomy and physiology of the muscle spindle in presented in Sections II and III. When we decided to update the text on the muscle spindle we determined that all the peripheral sensory receptors should be included. If you do not wish to include such information, Sections II and III can stand alone.

In order to facilitate the study of an admittedly overwhelming amount of material we recommend that you try to master one Section at a time. A summary of each major topic has been included to help you review the material. An index has been included for ease of reference.

Instructions

The information in this book is presented in a programmed learning format. It is important, however, for you to understand that this is not intended to be a true programmed text in that sufficient repetition for complete mastery of the subject in one reading is lacking. Additionally, more material may be presented in each frame than is tested in the blanks. The material has been designed primarily to allow the reader to interact with the broad range of subject matter in order to facilitate learning. It may be necessary, therefore, to proceed slowly, to read everything carefully and repeat each subsection in order to gain mastery of the material.

To proceed through the materials, begin with Stem 1. The answer will be found at the bottom and to the left of the question. You may wish to fold a piece of paper and cover the answers so you are not tempted to "peek" before committing yourself to an answer. The questions proceed in numerical order down the page. Turn the page to continue. Please note that a relatively long blank or blanks usually means a phrase of three or more words is required to answer the question.

SECTION I

The Motor Unit

1. The Motor Neuron
   a. The Cell body
   b. Axons and Terminal Branches

2. Muscle and Motor End Plates

3. Neuromuscular Junction

4. Functional Properties and Organization of Motor Units

5. Pathology and Mutability

THE MOTOR UNIT

1. A study of sensory receptors and sensory processing is not complete without some insight into the motor system. The motor system is the final common pathway for the expression of sensory input. Nervous system activity converges on this final pathway to produce or prevent a single event--muscle contraction.

    A detailed exploration of the anatomy and physiology of the motor system and its component parts will provide a better understanding of the function of specific sensory inputs which will be presented later in this text.

    We will begin, therefore, with components of the peripheral motor system. The peripheral motor system is composed of motor units which can be considered to be the elementary units of behavior in the skeletal motor system (Kandel, 1981).

    A motor unit is composed of (1) the motor neuron which consists of (a) the cell body, and (b) its axon and terminal branches; and (2) the neuromuscular junctions; and (3) all the muscle fibers (cells) that the neuron innervates.

    Label the diagram:

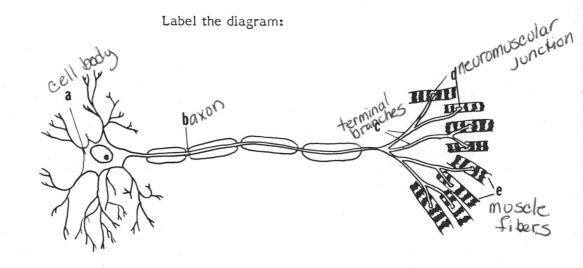

a. cell body
b. axon
c. terminal branches
d. neuromuscular junction
e. muscle fibers

2. In the normal state, the parts of a motor unit cannot be separated functionally. The entire unit responds in an "all or none" mode.

Whether the entire unit will respond is determined by the level of excitability in the cell body of the motor neuron.

The parts of the motor unit are:
(1) (a) _cell body_
    (b) _axon and branches_
(2) _neuromuscular junctions_ and
(3) _muscle fibers_

cell body
axon and branches
NMJ
muscle fibers

---

3. The motor neuron is often referred to as the anterior horn cell. It is so named because the cell bodies are located in the ventral or anterior horn of the grey matter of the spinal cord.

The anterior horn cell body receives input from the other nerve cells including interneurons in the spinal cord, from afferent axons, both direct and indirect via interneurons from the periphery, from the cortex and from other higher centers of the central nervous system.

This input determines the excitability level of the motor neuron. If the input is sufficient to activate the cell body, the motor unit will respond in an " _all-or-none_ " mode.

all-or-none

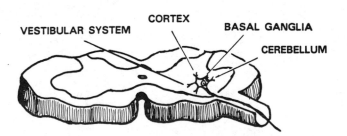

VESTIBULAR SYSTEM   CORTEX   BASAL GANGLIA   CEREBELLUM

4. When the motor neuron is activated the impulse is transmitted down the axon. This impulse triggers the release of transmitter substances which initiate changes in the permeability of the muscle cell membrane.

The resulting impulse or muscle action potential then sweeps the muscle fibers. The net result is contraction of all of the muscle fibers innervated by that one axon. Through this contraction we move our bony levers producing _motion_.

motion

---

5. Match the input and output labels with the appropriate structures.

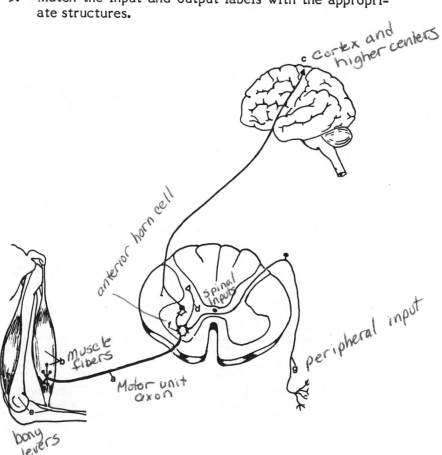

a. motor unit axon
b. muscle fibers
c. cortex & higher centers
d. spinal inputs
e. bony levers
f. anterior horn cell
g. peripheral input

5

6. All of the muscle fibers that are innervated by one neuron are homogenous or alike.

The "all or none" phenomenon refers to the response of the ___motor___ ___unit___.

motor unit

---

7. All of the muscle fibers that are contained in one motor unit are ___homogenous___.

homogenous or alike

---

8. The number of muscle fibers in a motor unit may vary from 2 or 3 to several thousand (Mountcastle, 1980). It is logical to conclude that the large motor units (those motor units which contain many muscle fibers) may be more involved in gross rather than fine movements.

Fine motor control, therefore, would be vested in motor units in which the innervation ratio is _____.

low or small

---

9. A motor unit which contains 500 muscle fibers would not likely be involved in _____ movements.

fine

---

10. The level of excitability of the motor neuron is determined by the _____ to it.

input

11. Motor units may be classified as being either phasic or tonic units according to their physiological properties. The terms phasic and tonic have come to mean many different things because of their use by different authors.

For the moment, we will consider "phasic" to mean fast or rapid muscle contraction. A tonic motor unit, on the other hand, will produce a slow, continuous muscle contraction.

Motor units may be functionally different from one another. In a more simplistic sense it could be said that an action such as hurling a javelin would strongly utilize motor units in the arm muscles that would be classified as _____ units.

phasic

---

12. The total tension that a given muscle can generate is determined by several factors. The most important of these factors are: (1) the number of muscle fibers activated and (2) the total tension produced by each muscle fiber.

The first factor is determined by the number of motor units recruited, and the number of muscle fibers per motor unit.

The second factor is determined by the frequency of the action potentials from the motor neuron and the characteristics of the muscle fibers themselves.

All of these components which are responsible for the total tension developed in a muscle will be explored throughout this book. For the present the most important factors in tension development are:
1) the number of _____ _____ activated;
2) the total tension produced by _____ _____ _____.

muscle fibers
each muscle fiber

13. The total tension developed in a given muscle is determined by: (1) the number of _____ _____ activated and (2) tension produced by each _____ _____.

muscle fibers
muscle fiber

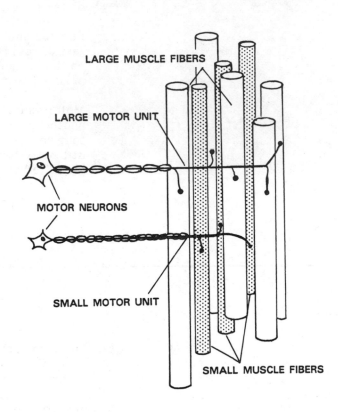

LARGE MUSCLE FIBERS

LARGE MOTOR UNIT

MOTOR NEURONS

SMALL MOTOR UNIT

SMALL MUSCLE FIBERS

14. The proper physiologic functioning of the motor unit as a whole depends upon the appropriate contributions of all the components of the motor unit. Each component has its own characteristics and functions within the unit.

A motor unit consists of the motor neuron, its communication with the muscle fibers via the neuromuscular junction, and the _____ fibers.

muscle

15. The entire motor unit responds by what has been described as the "_____" phenomenon.

all-or-none

_____

16. Diseases may affect different parts of the motor unit as well as the inputs the unit receives.

The level of excitability of the motor neuron is determined by the _____ it receives.

input

_____

17. The cell body of the motor neuron receives input from the _____, the _____ _____, and from _____ _____.

periphery
spinal cord
higher centers

_____

18. The amount and type of input to the motor neuron determines the level of neuronal _____.

excitability

_____

19. We may categorize motor units according to their physiological properties into at least two general categories: _____ and _____.

tonic
phasic

9

number of muscle
fibers activated

total tension produced
by **each** fiber

20. The most important factors in determining the total tension developed by a given muscle are:
(1) _____
and (2) _____.

---

large

21. Large movements or those requiring great muscle tension will be the responsibility of the motor units in which the innervation ratio of muscle fibers per axon is _____.

---

phasic
tonic

22. For the moment we may classify motor units functionally as either _____ or _____.

---

23. The motor unit functions as a result of the coordinated activity of its parts. Each component has its own characteristics and it is necessary to enumerate these characteristics before exploring the individual and collective actions of motor units as complete entities.

In the following sections we will look more closely at the individual characteristics of the components of the motor unit: 1) the _____, 2) the _____ and its terminal branches; the neuromuscular junctions and the _____ _____.

anterior horn cell body
axon
muscle fibers

10

SUMMARY

The motor unit is the smallest functional component of the neuromuscular system. It consists of the: (1) motor neuron which includes (a) the cell body and (b) its axon and terminal branches; (2) the neuromuscular junctions; and (3) all the muscle fibers which that neuron innervates.

This peripheral motor system is the final common pathway for the expression of sensory input. Nervous system activity converges on this final pathway to produce or prevent a single event--muscle contraction.

There is often confusion surrounding the labels given to the motor neuron. The motor neuron may be referred to as the anterior horn cell. Often the term "motor neuron" is used to refer to the cell body. To eliminate confusion the term is defined as follows:

> **Motor neuron** (anterior horn cell; alpha motor neuron)--the entire nerve cell including the cell body and its processes.

When the cell body of the motor neuron is excited to the threshold level the entire motor unit responds in an "all-or-nothing" mode.

The total tension a given muscle can generate is determined in large part by: (1) the total number of muscle fiber activated; and (2) the total tension produced by each muscle fiber.

Motor units may be functionally classified as **phasic** or **tonic,** and all of the muscle fibers in one motor unit are homogenous.

Motor units which contain many muscle fibers are activated when great levels of tension are required. Motor units with very few muscle fibers are largely responsible for fine, controlled movements.

The Cell Body

24. The cell bodies of motor neurons lie within the ventral horn of the spinal cord. We will look at some of their collective functions first and then explore the individual qualities and characteristics.

   The cell bodies of all the neurons which innervate a single muscle are referred to as a motor neuron pool. As you know, a given muscle such as the deltoid or biceps muscle will be supplied by neurons from two to four different segments of the spinal cord. Therefore, a motor neuron pool will span these different segments.

   In fact, a motor neuron pool will be organized longitudinally in a cell column (Kandel, 1981).

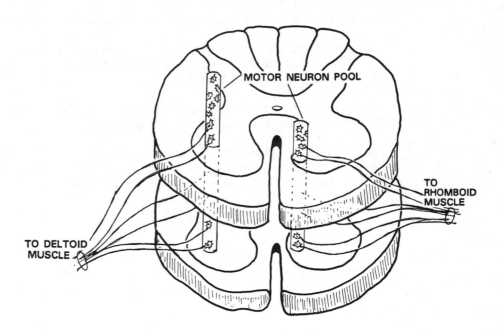

   A cell column making up a single motor neuron pool may span _____ spinal segments.

2-4

12

25. A motor neuron pool is designed for the single purpose of producing precise mechanical effects in its muscle (Henneman, 1980). To produce these effects and to operate under a wide variety of conditions the motor neuron pool must produce perfectly timed contractions of various numbers and types of its motor units.

The organization of the motor neuron pool must be understood if one is to understand some of the basic concepts of motor control.

The motor neuron pool is a functionally organized group of neurons which innervate a single _____.

muscle

26. The cell body is one part of the _____ _____.

motor neuron

27. A motor neuron pool is organized as a cell _____.

column

28. A motor neuron pool may span _____ spinal segments.

2-4

29. One motor neuron pool innervates _____ _____.

one muscle

30. As we just noted, the motor neuron pool consists of a group of cell bodies organized into vertical columns within the spinal cord. Motor neurons are also organized according to the areas of the body which they innervate.

Those motor neuron pools which innervate proximal muscles such as those of the neck and back are located medially. Those cells which innervate distal muscles such as those of the extremities and digits can be found in the dorsolateral part of the anterior horn.

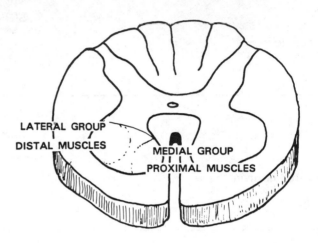

A motor neuron pool may span ____ spinal segments.

2-4

The motor neuron pool which innervates the flexor carpi radialis muscle is located in the _____ part of the ventral horn.

dorsolaterally

---

31. The lateral group of motor neuron pools is considerably larger than the medial group.

One could conclude, therefore, that those muscles which receive input from the largest group of motor neuron pools are the _____ muscles.

distal

14

32. Distal muscles are most likely to be involved in fine motor control. The number of muscle fibers in motor units of distal muscles may be relatively _____.

The number of motor neuron pools which innervate these motor units in distal muscles is _____.

small
large

---

33. Motor neuron pools are organized longitudinally in cell _____.

columns

---

34. One motor neuron pool innervates one specific _____.

muscle

---

35. The large lateral group of motor neuron pools innervates muscles of the _____.

extremities

---

36. Axial muscles of the neck and back are innervated by motor neuron pools in the _____ group.

medial

15

37. These pools are also organized according to their innervation of flexor or extensor muscle groups. Pools which innervate extensor muscles tend to lie ventral to those which innervate flexor muscles.

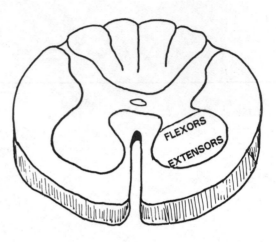

The most medial neuron pools innervate _____ muscles.

proximal

---

38. The most ventral motor neuron pools innervate _____ muscles.

extensor

---

39. Motor neuron pools innervating flexor muscles are located _____.

dorsally

would lie _____ and _____

ventrally
medially

41. Each of the motor neuron pools is arranged in a
_____ _____.

vertical column

---

42. Now that you have studied the general arrangement
of motor neurons as a group you will need to learn
the characteristics of **individual** motor neurons.
There are various sizes of cell bodies in a motor
neuron pool.

The largest motor neuron cell bodies may have as
much as 250,000 μm^2 of surface area and 10,000
synaptic knobs on their soma and dendrites. The
smallest may have as little as one twenty-fifth of
that surface area and correspondingly fewer synapses
(Mountcastle, 1980).

The largest motor neurons generally innervate the
greatest number of muscle fibers and therefore these
components comprise the _____ _____
units.

largest motor

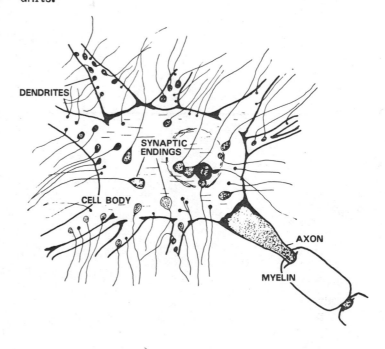

17

43. The electrical properties of motor neuron cell bodies also are related to their size. The smaller the cell body the more excitable it is because the threshold of activation is lower (Henneman, 1980).

Put another way, a lower intensity of stimulation is needed to discharge the _____ neurons.

smaller

---

44. The highest threshold of activation is found in the cell bodies of the _____ motor neurons.

largest

---

45. The susceptibility to inhibition also correlates with the size of the cell. The large cells are the easiest to inhibit and the small cells are the most difficult to inhibit (Harris and Henneman, 1979).

The susceptibility to inhibition is the reverse of that of activation. That is, the cells which are activated most easily are inhibited _____ easily.

least

---

46. Patterns of input to the motor neurons may also be different in large versus small cells and this may contribute to the correlation of size with excitability. We will consider this possibility later.

Another difference between small and large cells may be in the pattern of their _____.

input

47. Cell body size correlates strongly with excitability. A definite inverse relationship exists between cell size and the susceptibility to _____.

inhibition

---

48. The smallest cell bodies also have relatively long duration afterpotentials called afterhyperpolarization. As you know, any hyperpolarization of the cell membrane means that the membrane is made more difficult to depolarize or excite.

Long after-hyperpolarizations limit how rapidly the cell can be re-activated as a result of continued stimuli. Because of this property the small motor neurons fire at a lower frequency than the larger neurons. The initial threshold of activation, however, is lower in the small cells.

The threshold of activation and the maximum firing frequency of a motor neuron are two different characteristics. The small cells are most easily _____ and least easily _____.

activated
inhibited

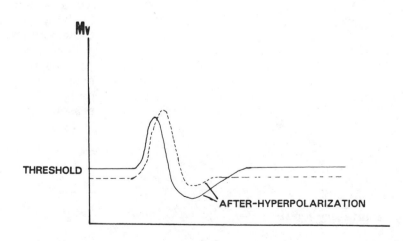

19

49. The small motor neurons fire at relatively lower _____ .

frequencies

---

50. Cell bodies of the large phasic motor neurons have a relatively short duration after-hyperpolarization and are, therefore, able to fire at very _____ frequencies (Bishop, 1982).

high

---

51. Motor neurons to the muscle cells are often referred to as **alpha** motor neurons. This name is derived from the size of the axons which are part of these neurons.

The motor neurons we have been studying may be called _____ motor neurons.

alpha

---

52. As a group, the alpha motor neurons are "lazy" (Bishop, 1982). That is, unlike some other neurons, these neurons do not spontaneously fire nor do they maintain some tonic activity level. Alpha motor neurons will discharge only when they are driven by excitatory inputs. Perhaps it is better to say these cells may be efficient in their function by only responding to an adequate input as opposed to being "lazy."

The only way to assure that an alpha motor neuron is going to be activated is to provide adequate _____ _____ .

excitatory input

53. Alpha motor neurons, however do have some compensatory qualities. For instance, when the depolarization is prolonged because of an above threshold stimulus the motor neuron will discharge repetitively.

In order to be activated, alpha motor neurons require _____ _____.

excitatory input

---

54. If, however, there is a prolonged depolarization from an above threshold stimulus the motor neuron will continue to _____.

fire or discharge

---

55. The maximal rate at which this continued firing occurs is dependent upon the duration of the after-potential that is characteristic of that cell.

The maximal firing rate would be the greatest in _____ motor neurons.

large

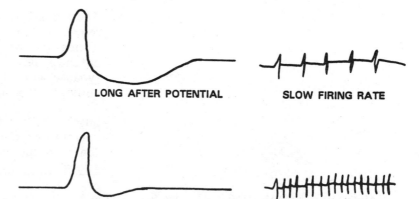

LONG AFTER POTENTIAL   SLOW FIRING RATE

SHORT AFTER POTENTIAL   FAST FIRING RATE

21

56. This ability to fire repetitively is a very important property of motor neurons. Repetitive firing provides a mechanism for coding neural input/output information. Functionally, this property is similar to that of sensory receptors which will be presented later in the appropriate sections of this text.

Input impulses are converted by the motor neuron cell bodies into output. If the intensity of the input is sufficient, the cell body will reach threshold and the entire cell will discharge.

The intensity of the input determines the rate of _____ _____.

repetitive firing
or
discharge

---

57. To review the concept of the all-or-none phenomenon (1) motor units are activated under the all-or-none law, (2) each synapse on the motor neurons produces graded responses which may or may not reach threshold and, therefore, do not follow the _____ law.

all-or-none

---

58. Another property of some central synapses, including some of those synapses that occur with the cell bodies of motor neurons, is that of post-tetanic potentiation. Following a rapid repetitive input the synapse will experience a long lasting increase in its ability to transmit.

Susceptibility to post-tetanic potentiation is also correlated to cell size (Bishop, 1982). The small tonic motor neurons are the most susceptible to _____ _____.

post-tetanic potentiation

22

transmit
or
discharge

59. With post-tetanic potentiation a fast repetitive input to the synapse will result in a long-lasting increase in its ability to _____.

---

60. This property of post-tetanic potentiation (PTP) has functional implications to be considered later. PTP will also be encountered in the discussion on muscle.

Maintained and repetitive use of synapses will alter their efficiency. Alteration in activity because of repetitive activation may ultimately result in actual changes in the function of a synapse.

For the moment, it is only necessary to understand that those motor neurons which are the most susceptible to post-tetanic potentiation are the _____ neurons.

small

---

61. Some of the properties of motor neurons which correlate with their size may appear to be contradictory. All the properties of the motor neuron which relate to its size, however, contribute to the overall functioning of the cell.

The small motor neurons have the lowest threshold to activation, and are the least susceptible to inhibition. Also, these cells have the longest after-hyperpolarization and, therefore, the slowest firing rate.

You have just learned that the small cells are also the most susceptible to _____ _____.

post-tetanic potentiation

62. These may sound like opposite functions, but let's look at it another way. The small motor units cannot be activated at a high firing rate, but they can maintain their activity for long periods of time. Thus, PTP will be most effective with such long enduring cells.

Cells that will be maintaining activity for long periods of time should also have low thresholds so they will be activated first. Cells that fatigue rapidly should only be called in when absolutely required for high frequency, high tension responses so they will have _____ thresholds.

high

---

63. The motor neurons which are the least susceptible to post-tetanic potentiation are the _____ ones.

largest

---

64. Motor neurons may also be classified as to "critical firing level" (Henneman & Mendell, 1981) which is similar in concept to the term "threshold" but defined somewhat differently. The term critical firing level has also been used to describe the percent of active excitatory inputs upon a single motor neuron necessary for an action potential to be generated. In the following discussion the term will be used to describe a recruitment order.

Consider the total number of motor neuron cell bodies in a pool innervating a muscle. If all the neurons are activated, then that obviously represents 100 percent of the pool. If we record from one cell body in that pool we can see when it is activated relative to all the other neurons.

Thus the critical firing level of a single neuron may be defined as a percentage of the total output of the motor neuron _____.

pool

24

65. One neuron may be activated at the point when 60 percent of the cell bodies are active. Another may come in at the 45 percent level and so forth. The critical firing level of a neuron appears to remain constant. That is, it always comes in when 60 percent of the cell bodies are active. At 58 percent activation it is silent.

It has been noted that there may be an uncertain zone of approximately 2 percent (Henneman & Mendell, 1981). That is, the exact critical firing level of a neuron may vary as much as 2 percent. In the example above, the neuron may fire at the 59 percent level or perhaps not until 61 percent of the cell bodies have been _____.

activated

---

66. The critical firing level of a neuron remains constant in relation to the other neurons in the pool. Even if the critical firing level of two neurons are very close together such as 35.6 percent versus 36 percent the former will most likely be activated before the latter.

The critical firing level of a particular motor neuron cell body may be defined as a percentage of the total output of the _____ _____ _____.

motor neuron pool

---

67. The motor neurons with the lowest "critical firing level" are the most responsive during any mono-synaptic reflex recording. They are also the most responsive to repetitive firing.

No matter how the motor neuron is activated the one that is most responsive is the one with the _____ level.

lowest critical firing

68. As you might expect, those neurons with the lowest critical firing levels are the smallest ones. They are also served by the smallest axons.

The critical firing level appears to be highly correlated with cell _____.

size

---

69. Cells which are the most susceptible to both monosynaptic reflexes and repetitive firing are the _____ cells.

small

---

70. Before considering the properties of the axons of the motor neurons, a review of the properties of individual and groups of motor neuron cell bodies will help lessen your confusion and enhance your progress in studying the other components of the motor unit.

All the cell bodies of neurons which supply a given muscle are contained in a _____ _____.

motor neuron pool

---

71. A motor neuron pool is organized _____ and may span _____ segments.

longitudinally
2-4

72. Within the ventral horn of the spinal cord, the cell bodies of those motor neuron pools which innervate proximal muscles such as those of the neck and back are located _____.

medially

---

73. Relative to those motor neurons which innervate extensor muscles, the motor neuron pools in the ventral horn which innervate flexor muscles are located _____.

dorsally

---

74. The motor neuron pools which innervate distal muscles such as those of the extremities are located _____.

laterally

---

75. In terms of size, compared to the medial group of motor neuron pools, the lateral group is the _____.

largest

---

76. The most excitable cells, or those with the lowest threshold of activation, are the _____ cells.

smallest

27

77. The largest cells are the _____ to inhibit.

easiest

---

78. Another difference between large and small cells may be in the pattern of their _____.

input

---

79. Those cells with the longest duration after hyperpolarization and, therefore, the lowest maximum frequency are the _____ cells.

small

---

80. The cells which are least susceptible to post-tetanic potentiation are the _____ cells.

large

---

81. Alpha motor neurons require excitatory input in order to be _____.

driven or activated

---

82. The smallest cells are the most difficult to _____.

inhibit

83. If there is a prolonged depolarization of a cell it will
_____ _____.

fire repetitively

___

84. The "critical firing level" of a single motor neuron is defined as a percentage of the total output of the
_____ _____ _____.

motor neuron pool

___

85. Consider the neuron that has a critical firing level such that it always fires when 35.6 percent of the pool has been activated. Another cell may have a critical firing level of 36 percent. Therefore, the first cell described will most likely be activated _____ the last cell.

before

___

86. Large neurons have the _____ critical firing level.

highest

___

87. Repetitive use of synapses will alter the efficiency of those synapses. Continued activity may ultimately result in actual changes in the structure and _____ of a synapse.

function

88. There may be additional differences in motor neurons which are worth considering. It has been assumed that a motor neuron pool contains cells that differ only by their sizes. There is newer evidence that there are different types of cells in each pool. The only characteristic other than size that has been identified and measured, however, is the cell's rate of firing (Mountcastle, 1980).

In a study of the motor neuron pool supplying the plantaris muscle of cats, cell bodies of the same size were found to fire at rates which varied as much as two to three times.

There is evidence, therefore, that all cells of the same size may not have the same _____ _____.

firing rate

---

89. In addition, there is evidence to suggest that inhibitory inputs may affect different types of cells in a different manner.

Remember that these different **types** of cells may be found among cells of the same _____.

size

---

90. Relative to cell size, the input resistance (the electrical resistance between the inside and outside of the cell) to a motor neuron is inversely proportional to the size of the cell as defined by the somatic surface area of the cell.

A high input resistance means that the electrical charge will spread more rapidly **inside** the membrane and thus produce a **larger** excitatory potential.

The input resistance to the larger cells would be _____ than that to the small cells.

lower

91. Although input resistance may be one of the most important factors in determining the critical firing level of a cell, a number of other properties that we know little about may contribute to such phenonema.

Some other properties which may differ and may be correlated with cell type or size are: specific resistance per unit area, density of sodium gates and cell geometry (Henneman, 1980).

Studies suggest that the differences between the cells lie within the cells themselves.

Some researchers have suggested that the differences between cells may be due to differences in inputs to the cells. The above evidence indicates the differences are more likely to be within the _____.

cells

---

92. The "critical firing level" of any particular motor neuron has been defined as a percentage. Thus, this level in any one neuron is expressed in relation to _____.

all the other neurons in the motor neuron pool

---

93. The differences between cells have primarily been described relative to different _____ of the cells.

sizes

---

94. It has also been noted that some differences may exist between cells of the _____ _____.

same size

31

SUMMARY

The motor unit is the fundamental unit of neuromuscular function and consists of the neuron (cell body, axon and terminal branches) along with the neuromuscular junctions and all the muscle fibers innervated by that one neuron. The motor unit is activated in an all-or-none fashion.

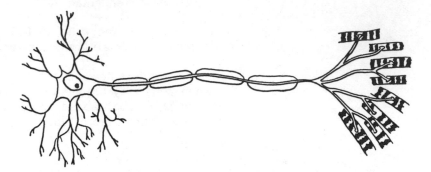

All the cell bodies of motor neurons which innervate a given muscle are organized together in a longitudinal column which spans several spinal cord levels. This collection of cells is referred to as the motor neuron pool.

If the motor neuron pools are considered collectively, the large lateral group innervates muscles of the extremities. The medial group innervates proximal muscles such as those of the neck and back. The pools can also be grouped dorsally and ventrally, the former innervating flexors and the latter the extensors.

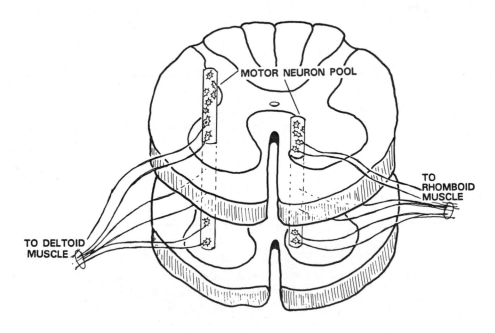

The cell bodies of alpha motor neurons have a number of characteristics which are strongly correlated with size. They are summarized in the following chart:

Small Cell Bodies	Large Cell Bodies
Easiest to activate	Highest threshold of activation
Least susceptible to inhibition	Most susceptible to inhibition
Longest after hyperpolarization	Shortest after hyperpolarization
Slowest maximum firing rate	Highest firing rate or frequency
Most susceptible to post-tetanic potentiation	Least susceptible to post-tetanic potentiation
Lowest critical firing level	Highest critical firing level
Most susceptible to mono-synaptic reflexes	Less susceptible to monosynaptic reflexes
High input resistance	Lower input resistance

The critical firing level of the motor neuron may determine its order of recruitment and is relatively stable in relation to all the other motor neurons in the pool. The critical firing level is expressed as a percentage of active motor neurons in a pool. If a neuron is activated when 35 percent of the neurons in the pool are active, the critical firing level is 35 percent.

Evidence also suggests that there are differences between cells which are not related to cell size. There are different types of cells found among those of the same size.

95. The axon, of course, is the part of the motor neuron which carries any generated electrical pulse to another nerve cell or to the effector organ such as muscle. The axon is the longest of the cell's processes.

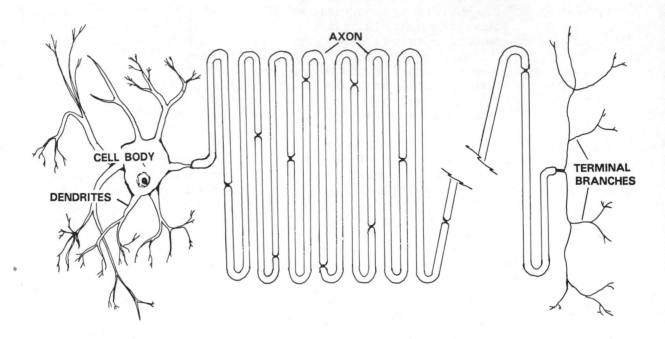

The axon is much like an electrical cable. If a threshold stimulus is reached an action potential is generated. The axon is capable of regenerating or propagating action potentials along its length. If this were not so, an electric signal would be carried passively only a very short distance along the axon.

It will not be the purpose of this text to review all the electric properties of axons and other excitable membranes. There are definite differences among axons which mostly relate to their diameter and such membrane properties as resistance and capacitance. These differences will only be summarized here. The reader is referred to any good physiology text for a more detailed insight into these properties.

The axon must be capable of propagating an _____ _____.

action potential

96. Most of the differences among peripheral axons may be summarized as being the result of axonal _____ and inherent _____ properties.

diameter
membrane

---

97. The largest diameter axons have the fastest _____ _____.

conduction velocities

---

98. The largest axons have the heaviest myelin sheaths which also contribute to the fast _____ _____.

conduction velocities

MYELIN SHEATH

35

99. As you might now expect, the largest axons have the lowest threshold to electrical stimulation. This size characteristic is completely opposite to the sensitivity of the cell body.

In other words, the large axons have low thresholds but their cell bodies have _____ thresholds.

high

---

100. The largest axons also produce the _____ action potentials.

largest

---

101. The smallest axons: (choose one)

   a) have the (largest/smallest) radius
   b) have the (fastest/slowest) conduction velocity
   c) have the (heaviest/lightest) coat of myelin
   d) have the (highest/lowest) threshold to electrical stimulation
   e) produce the (highest/lowest) amplitude action potentials

a. smallest
b. slowest
c. lightest
d. highest
e. lowest

---

102. The function of the axon is much like that of an electrical cable. In order to transmit information from one place to another it must be able to regenerate _____ _____ throughout its length.

action potentials

103. Because of anatomic and physiologic differences, axons have different functional properties. Temperature affects the conduction velocity of axons. The smallest axons are slowly blocked with a decrease in temperature, however, large fibers are rapidly blocked by such temperature reduction.

In comparison to the smaller axons, blocking or slowing the conduction in the largest axon requires a _____ drop in temperature.

smaller

---

104. Large axons are also more susceptible to ischemia. Externally applied pressure produces a local ischemia which will affect conduction of the large axons more readily than smaller axons.

The smaller axons will be resistant to pressure blocks while transmission of large axons can be effectively blocked by locally applied _____.

pressure

---

105. Small axons, on the other hand, are more susceptible to certain local anesthetics. It would seem that blocking one size of fiber would be quite possible with either of the previously named mechanisms or substances.

It is not possible to get a pure block of a particular sensation or function, however, because the different receptors and motor cell bodies have overlapping sizes of axons.

As you will remember, the largest motor neurons have the _____ axons.

largest

37

106. The motor neurons are sometimes referred to as alpha motor neurons. This name relates to the size of the axon. Motor neurons may be referred to as anterior horn cells and _____ motor neurons.

alpha

107. The largest axons are most susceptible to a change in _____.

temperature

108. The smallest axons are least susceptible to pressure which produces a local _____.

ischemia

109. Local anesthetics have the greatest effect on the _____ axons.

small

110. One might wish to be completely selective when attempting to block a group of particular size fibers utilizing the mechanism or substances noted.

Such selectivity is not possible because _____ _____.

cells with different functions have an overlap in the size of their axons

111. Along its course the axon may give off branches. These are termed axon collaterals. If this branching occurs in alpha motor neurons it would be called an alpha _____.

collateral

---

112. At its terminus, the axon may divide into few or many terminal branches. These are the branches that will innervate each of the muscle fibers in the motor unit.

The largest axons will have the _____ branches.

most

---

113. The action potential that is generated in the axon is transmitted faithfully in all its collaterals and _____ branches.

terminal

114. The axon is connected to the cell body by the initial segment. The initial segment has the lowest threshold of any part of the axon. It serves as the passive summing point for the synaptic currents generated within the cell body. It is, therefore, considered to be the trigger zone of the neuron.

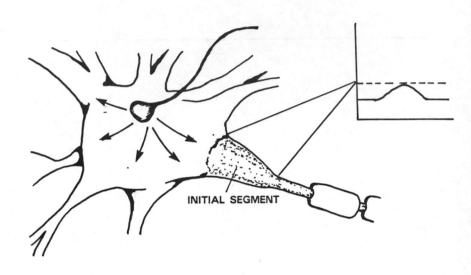

INITIAL SEGMENT

Whether the currents generated in the cell body are to be propagated along the axon is determined by the level of excitability in the _____.

initial segment

---

115. The threshold of the initial segment determines the level of excitability of the entire axon. The initial segment is located in the area at which the _____ joins the _____.

axon
cell body

SUMMARY

Small Diameter Axons

Slower conduction velocity
Smallest myelin coat
Highest threshold to electrical
   stimulation
Produces smallest amplitude
   action potential
Resistant to temperature
   changes
Resistent to ischemia
Susceptible to local anesthetics

Large Diameter Axons

Faster conduction velocity
Heaviest myelin coat
Lowest threshold to electrical
   stimulation
Produces highest amplitude
   action potential
Susceptible to temperature
   changes
Susceptible to ischemia
Resistant to local anesthetics

Action potentials propagated along the axon will be faithfully reproduced
in all collaterals and terminal branches.

The initial segment of the axon has the lowest threshold and is considered
to be the trigger zone of the neuron.

116. When discussing muscle it is necessary to differenti-
ate between a muscle cell, a muscle unit and a
muscle.

The muscle cell is often called the muscle fiber and
it is the smallest functional division of a muscle. A
skeletal muscle such as the brachialis is composed of
many muscle cells.

A "muscle unit" is a term used to refer to all the
muscle cells in a given motor unit. All muscle cells
in a muscle unit are _____.

homogenous
or
alike

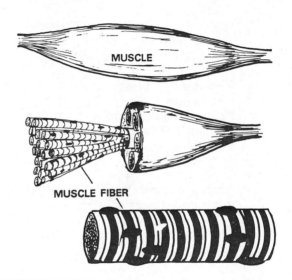

MUSCLE

MUSCLE FIBER

117. A single neuron with all the muscle fibers it
innervates is called a _____ _____.

motor unit

118. All muscle cells in a motor unit are referred to as the
_____ _____.

muscle unit

119. The muscle cell consists of an excitable cell membrane, the sarcolemma, and a repeated pattern of contractile elements. Of course, the cell has mitochondria and other cellular organelles just as do other types of cells. Each muscle cell is composed of many myofibirils which are made up of repeating patterns of contractile proteins. This repeated pattern gives the cell its banded or striated appearance.

You will remember that the smallest contractile unit in the myofibrils is the sarcomere. Each sarcomere consists of a number of bands which are light and dark in relation to one another. These bands show the arrangement of contractile proteins within the _____.

sarcomere

MUSCLE FIBER

I BAND   A BAND

MYOFIBRIL

SARCOMERE

ACTIN FILAMENT

MYOSIN FILAMENT

ACTIN MOLECULES   MYOSIN MOLECULES

120. That there was more than one type of muscle cell was apparent as long ago as 1874 when Ranvier observed that mammalian skeletal muscles differed in color and microscopic appearance. The smaller fibers were darker in color and were thus described as "red". The larger fibers were light in color and were described as "_____."

white

---

121. Muscle fibers may be called red and white from a gross observational perspective, and also on the basis of contractile speed.

Early experiments with electrical stimulation showed a difference in contractile properties of muscle fibers. With the advent of advanced technology, however, at least **three** types of fibers have been identified in mammalian muscle (Edgerton, 1976; Mountcastle, 1980; Bishop, 1982).

Because the research which involves muscle fiber typing has been done by different laboratories, each emphasizing different aspects of the structure or function of the muscle cells, there are many different names for these three types of cells.

Muscle fibers have been classified by Brooke (1971) as to types I and II. The white muscle fibers may be subdivided into two categories: type IIA and IIB. The type IIA fiber is often classified as an intermediate fiber.

Red fibers may be referred to as type _____ fibers.

I

---

122. Red and white muscle fibers may be classified as to contractile speed. Red fibers are relatively slow to react to a stimulus and white fibers will react _____.

quickly or rapidly

123. Muscle cells derive their energy from utilizing oxygen or by hydrolyzing glycogen. Muscle samples may be stained histochemically for the enzymes utilized in their metabolism. The type I fibers stain darkly when tested for oxidative enzymes.

The white fibers stain as follows: type IIA have both oxidative and glycolytic enzymes. The type IIB stains darkly when examined for glycolytic enzymes.

Based on this information, one could label the intermediate fiber as type _____.

IIA

---

124. Combining enzyme and contractile characteristics, muscle fibers have been labeled as **SO**--slow oxidative; **FOG**--fast oxidative glycolytic, and; **FG**--fast _____ (Peter, et.al., 1972).

glycolytic

---

125. Muscle cells which are rich in oxidative enzymes are the type _____ fibers.

I

---

126. The FOG fiber may be considered the same as type _____.

IIA

---

127. Type I fibers have also been labeled as _____.

SO

45

128. When examined for endurance characteristics muscle cells have been labeled **S**--slow and unfatiguable; **FR**--fast fatigue resistant; and **FF**--fast fatiguable (Burke, 1967; 1971; 1973).

The speed of contraction of type I muscle fibers is _____.

slow

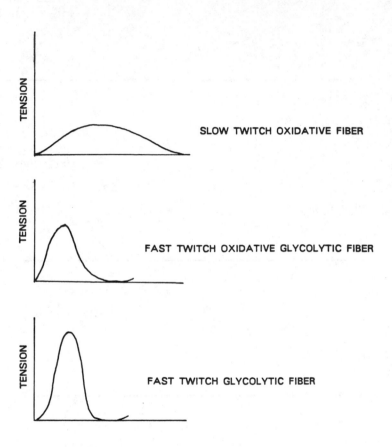

SLOW TWITCH OXIDATIVE FIBER

FAST TWITCH OXIDATIVE GLYCOLYTIC FIBER

FAST TWITCH GLYCOLYTIC FIBER

129. Look at the diagram above. The fiber with the greatest peak tension is the _____ fiber.

IIB

130. These three classification systems may be more easily visualized in table form:

Red	Intermediate	White
I	IIA	IIB
SO	FOG	FG
S	FR	FF

Because there are different criteria for these classifications it may not be totally accurate to assume that all three classifications are equivalent and represent the same muscle fibers (Rose and Rothstein, 1983). That is, fibers identified as type I, SO and S may not actually be the same fiber. Nonetheless, it will serve our purposes to assume that they are equivalent.

For our purposes we can say that the intermediate type of muscle fibers may also be referred to as type _____, _____ and _____.

IIA
FOG
FR

---

131. Fast fatiguable muscle fibers (type IIB) are specialized for the production of energy (ATP) by glycolysis and are, therefore, referred to as _____ fibers.

glycolytic

---

132. The muscle fibers which utlize oxygen in their metabolic cycle contract _____ and do not _____ readily.

slowly
fatigue

133. The metabolic enzymes in type I muscle fibers which synthesize ATP require the presence of _____.

oxygen

TYPE I FIBERS   TYPE IIA FIBERS   TYPE IIB FIBERS

TYPE IIA FIBERS STAIN WITH BOTH ENZYME STAINS

OXDATIVE ENZYME STAIN

GLYCOLYTIC ENZYME STAIN

BOTH STAINS

---

134. Two investigators have described at least one more fiber type, possibly two. Very little is known about these types and, if present, they appear to make up a very small percentage of the total muscle (Brooke & Kaiser, 1970; Burke, 1980).

We will consider the number of muscle fiber types to be _____ in number.

three

---

135. The variety of labels for these three muscle cell types has been the result of fiber typing by different laboratories which emphasize different aspects of muscle cell structure and _____.

function

48

136. The three types of fibers differ in many characteristics such as number and arrangement of organelles, capillary density associated with the fibers and specific types of contractile proteins. A partial table of differences is presented. Using the table answer the questions which follow.

Characteristics of Muscle Fiber Types

Type I (SO, S)	Type IIA (FOG, FR)	Type IIB (FG, FF)
Red	White	White
Slow twitch	Fast twitch	Fast twitch
Unfatiguable	Fatigue resistant	Fatiguable
Aerobic	Aerobic, anaerobic	Anaerobic
Small fiber	Intermediate fiber	Large fiber
Low peak tension	Intermediate peak tension	High peak tension

The fiber type with the most mitochondria is the _____.

I (SO, S)

The fiber type which utilizes oxygen metabolism (aerobic) is the _____.

I (SO, S)

Increased capillary density is associated with the need for _____.

oxygen

The fiber type which utilizes glycogen (anaerobic) in its metabolism is _____.

IIB (FG, FF)

The largest fiber is the _____.

IIB (FG, FF)

The fiber which can utilize both oxygen and glycogen is the _____.

IIA (FOG, FR)

137. The biochemical pathways producing ATP which is utilized during muscle contraction is illustrated below.

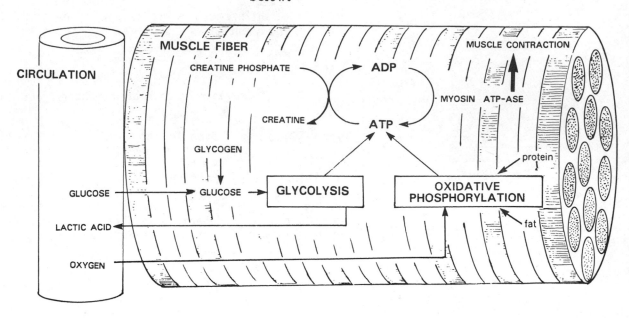

The speed with which a muscle fiber contracts depends upon how fast it can split ATP. The myosin-ATPase activity is the highest in type _____ fibers.

II

---

138. Fibers which produce lactic acid as a by-product of metabolism are the type _____ fibers.

II

---

139. The muscle fibers which can metabolize fat and protein are primarily the type _____ fibers.

I

---

140. The major source of phosphate found in the muscle cells which is utilized in the production of ATP is the compound _____ _____.

creatine phosphate

141. Type I muscle fibers have a slow speed of contraction. They generate a relatively small amount of tension. These muscle fibers are very resistant to fatigue and function in the presence of oxygen.

Type I muscle fibers function with _____ metabolism.

aerobic or oxygen

142. Type IIA muscle fibers have a fast speed of contraction. They are intermediate in the amount of tension they can develop. These fibers also are resistant to fatigue.

Type IIA muscle fibers use both _____ and _____ metabolism.

anaerobic, aerobic

143. Type IIB muscle fibers have a fast speed of contraction. They generate a large amount of tension. These fibers fatigue rapidly and function in the absence of oxygen.

Type IIB muscle fibers function through _____ metabolism.

anaerobic

144. The muscle fibers which generate a relatively low peak tension but may be able to sustain contractions indefinitely are the type _____ fibers.

I

145. Although the speed of contraction of a muscle depends on the type of enzyme activity, the total tension developed at any one cross bridge is the same for all types. The total tension in the fiber depends on the number of cross bridges that are active (Vander, et.al., 1980).

The largest cell will have the most myofilaments so it also has the most cross bridges active and therefore will be capable of generating the most _____.

tension

---

146. The type of enzyme activity determines the fiber's susceptibility to fatigue as well as its speed of contraction. The fibers which utilize oxygen metabolism are the _____ fatiguable.

least

---

147. Fill in the following table:

	Type I	Type IIA	Type IIB
speed of contraction			
tension development			
rate of fatigue			
fiber size			

check with
Table on
page 50

---

148. Muscle fibers which will be innervated by the largest motor neurons are the type _____ fibers.

IIB

149. It is easy to see the value of the above differences among fibers. Some functional activities require the maintainance of muscle contraction for long periods of time without fatigue. This is particularly true of the postural muscles.

Arm muscles may have to produce large amounts of tension rapidly for activities such as lifting or throwing. Obviously many activities require both kinds of ability.

Running a marathon would require primarily type _____ muscle fibers.

I

---

150. In lower animals a given muscle may be homogenous. For example, the soleus may consist entirely of type I fibers while the fast gastrocnemius will be composed entirely of type II fibers.

In man, however, there is a mixture of all three muscle fiber types in every muscle. Different fiber types may predominate in various muscles in the same person.

Additionally, a certain muscle in one individual may have predominately type I fibers while the same muscle in another individual may have more type __ fibers.

II

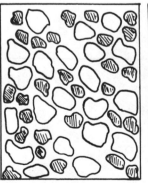 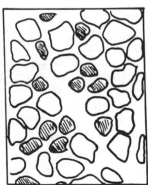

TYPE I FIBERS
IN
SUBJECT A

TYPE I FIBERS
IN
SUBJECT B

151. Perhaps the most important property of muscle cells is their mutability or the ability to undergo change. Muscle adapts very well to the different demands placed upon it.

This is why as therapists, we design different types of exercise training programs to suit the patient's needs.

The most important property of muscle may be its ability to undergo _____.

change

---

152. Muscle is a very dynamic tissue. If a lengthened position is maintained it adapts by adding sarcomeres.

If the muscle is maintained in a shortened position it adapts by _____ _____.

subtracting
or
losing sarcomeres

---

153. Experiments and observations of muscle tissue response to stresses, positions or other forms of manipulation, show that such changes can begin within 12 hours.

One way to maintain a muscle at a particular length for 12 hours or more would be to apply a _____ to the associated joints.

cast
or
brace

---

154. Muscle is altered in the presence of primary muscle diseases such as muscular dystrophy.

Even more important to the field of rehabilitation is the finding that muscle is altered in response to normal and abnormal stresses and diseases of other systems as well.

The structure and function of the muscle fibers may occur in the presence of spasticity and other manifestations of disorders of the _____ system.

nervous

SUMMARY

Muscle cells or fibers may be classified into three types based on differences in many characteristics of structure and function. There may be other types of fibers, however, they are not considered in this text.

Characteristics of Muscle Fiber Types

Type I (SO, S)	Type IIA (FOG, FR)	Type IIB (FG, FF)
Red	White	White
Slow twitch	Fast twitch	Fast twitch
Unfatiguable	Fatigue resistant	Fatiguable
Aerobic	Aerobic, anaerobic	Anaerobic
Small fiber	Intermediate fiber	Large fiber
Low peak tension	Intermediate peak tension	High peak tension

The most important property of muscle may be its mutability--the ability to undergo change. Patients with central nervous system disorders often experience further impairment in motor function as a result of changes in muscle itself (Tabary, et.al., 1981).

Muscle tissue is altered when subjected to alterations in input such as with spasticity or rigidity. Muscle tissue responds to positions or conditions which result in a lengthened or shortened state. It is affected by exercise and disuse and, of course, by primary diseases of muscle.

155. The neuromuscular junction or motor end plate area is pictured below.

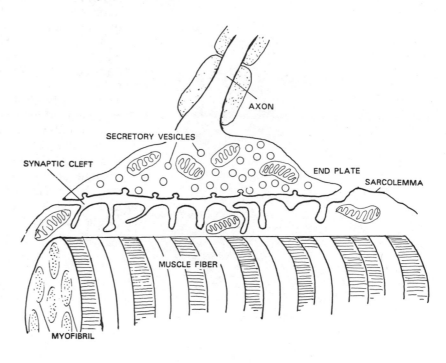

The neuromuscular junction (NMJ) is the structure which allows communication between the _____ and the _____.

axon
muscle

---

156. It is not necessary to enumerate all the variations in the motor end plate complex. It is useful to know that there are three distinct types of neuromuscular junctional complexes - one for each muscle fiber type.

The neuromuscular junctional complexes are correlated with differences in susceptibility to neuromuscular fatigue.

Each muscle fiber type has its own unique _____ junction.

neuromuscular

157. It is possible to summarize briefly the activities which occur at the neuromuscular junction (NMJ) relative to neuromuscular transmission.

A nerve impulse which has been propagated along the axon from the cell body, invades and depolarizes all of the nerve terminals. This action produces a calcium ion influx which causes the secretory vesicles to release the neurotransmitter, acetylcholine.

The acetylcholine molecules which have been released diffuse across the synaptic cleft to bind to acetylcholine receptors on the post-synaptic membrane. The transmitter receptor complex induces a change in the conformation of the membrane. This change opens channels to ionic flow and the muscle cell is depolarized. The potential which is produced at the NMJ is called the end-plate potential (EPP) (Mountcastle, 1980; Vander, et.al., 1980).

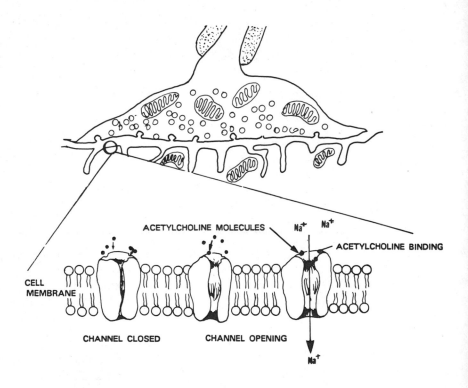

Calcium ions cause the release of neurotransmiter from the _____ _____.

secretory vesicles

158. Under normal conditions the amplitude of the end-plate potential is large enough to trigger a muscle action potential. This is the only known synapse in which one presynaptic impulse produces one post-synaptic impulse. This phenomenon accounts for the all-or-none nature of the firing of the motor unit.

Multiple inputs are necessary to activate the motor neuron cell body sufficiently to depolarize the initial segment, yet only one input is necessary to activate the _____ cells.

muscle

---

159. The muscle membrane systems and neuromuscular junctional complexes of each of the three types of muscle cells are uniquely structured to that particular cell.

The unique structures contribute to the different qualities of muscle cell physiology such as contractile speed and the speed with which the action potential sweeps the muscle cell (Mountcastle, 1980).

The speed of the action potential is partially determined by the different qualities of the _____ junctions.

neuromuscular

---

160. You will recall the discussion of the phenomenon of post-tetanic potentiation (PTP) in relation to some central synapses. We said that the motor neuron cell bodies which were most susceptible to PTP were the _____ cells.

small

161. Post-tetanic potentiation also occurs at the NMJ after a short period of high frequency repetitive stimulation. This facilitation can last for several minutes.

The muscle fibers which are most susceptible to PTP are the slow, fatigue resistant fibers. These are the _____ (largest/smallest) muscle fibers.

smallest

---

162. The property of post-tetanic potentiation creates a prolonged facilitation following a _____ _____ stimulus.

fast repetitive

---

163. PTP occurs at synapes on both the motor neuron cell body and the muscle cell. In both cases, the cells most susceptible to post-tetanic potentiation are the _____ cells.

smaller

THRESHOLD CHANGES WITH PTP

---

164. Large motor neurons are the least susceptible to _____ _____.

post-tetanic potentiation

165. There are some other interesting forms of facilitation which may be of use clinically. Stretch of the muscle cells results in an augmented release of ACh which increases the amplitude of the end-plate potential (EPP).

The deformation caused by the mechanical stretch in some way releases a larger number of vesicles of _____.

acetylcholine

---

166. Investigators have described an increase in tension of a fatigued skeletal muscle by activation of the sympathetic fibers innervating it (Hutter and Lowenstein, 1955).

Epinephrine and norepinephrine produce increased tension. These agents produced by stimulation of the sympathetic nerves and organs associated with sympathetic nervous system activation result in an increased amplitude of the end plate potential produced by the motor nerve impulse.

Sympathetic nervous system activation produces an increase in the amplitude of the _____.

EPP

---

167. Three ways in which muscle fiber activation may be facilitated are (1) _____ _____, (2) _____ _____, and (3) activation of the _____.

1. mechanical stretch
2. repetitive activation
3. sympathetic nervous system

SUMMARY

The neuromuscular junction is a specialized structure which allows the impulse from the neuron to activate the muscle cell so it can produce a contraction.

There are at least three distinct neuromuscular junctional complexes—one for each muscle fiber type.

The neuromuscular junction is the only known synapse in which one presynaptic impulse produces one post-synaptic impulse. In motor neurons one synapse is not sufficient to produce a post-synaptic impulse.

Post-tetanic potentiation is a property of the NMJ just as it was in certain central synapses. After a period of high frequency repetitive stimulation a prolonged facilitation occurs. Cells which are most susceptible to PTP are the smaller cells.

Ways in which muscle fibers can be facilitated are through mechanical stretch, repetitive activation and activation of the sympathetic nervous system.

Full-blown activation of the sympathetic nervous system results in mobilization of the musculature in a fight or flight response. Such a response can be elicited from pain, anger, excitement, and noxious stimuli, to name a few. Milder levels of activation of the sympathetic nervous system may follow the same types of stimuli usually of a less severe or threatening quality.

168. Initially, you studied the anatomical organization of the motor unit. You have just spent considerable time investigating the anatomy and physiology of the various components of the motor unit.

Now it would seem appropriate to put the parts together again and consider some functional properties of the motor unit as a whole.

The motor unit consists of the (1)_____, (2)_____, (3)_____, (4)_____ and all the _____ _____ it innervates.

cell body
axon
terminal branches
NMJ
muscle fibers

---

169. Motor units are usually labeled according to the muscle units involved. So, among others, we could label the motor units as type I, _____ and _____.

type IIA
type IIB

---

170. Fill in the chart:

MOTOR UNIT TYPES

	I	IIA	IIB
Motor neuron cell size	small	intermediate	_____
Critical firing level	earliest	intermediate	latest
Susceptibility to inhibition	least	intermediate	greatest
Susceptibility to post-tetanic potentiation	greatest	intermediate	least
Duration of hyperpolarization after-potentials	longest	intermediate	_____
Axons			
cross-sectional area	smallest	intermediate	_____
conduction velocity	slowest	intermediate	_____
NMJ Type	I	IIA	IIB
Susceptibility to PTP	greatest	intermediate	least
Muscle fibers			
size	smallest	intermediate	largest
fatiguability	least	intermediate	_____
speed of contraction	slowest	intermediate	_____
maximal tension	lowest	intermediate	_____
oxygen system	yes	yes	no
glycolytic	no	yes	yes
Consequence of activity	slow, gross, posture movements	fast	rapid, precise phasic movement

large
shortest
largest
fastest
most
fastest
highest

63

171. So you can see that, for the most part, the various components of the motor unit are "matched up" -- that is, the large, high-threshold cells have large, fast-conducting axons which innervate large, fast-contracting muscle fibers. The largest number of these fibers are found in the IIB unit.

Thus we have a high threshold, rapidly contracting, high tension-generating motor unit which produces rapid and high tension output movements.

Write out the same description for a type I motor unit.

Low threshold, slowly contacting,
low tension-generating motor unit
which produces slow, gross,
postural movements.

---

172. One method of recruitment is the activation of increasingly greater numbers of motor neurons. Recruitment of motor units was mentioned earlier as the method of increasing the total tension in a muscle.

Total tension depends upon the total number of motor units recruited and the size of the units that are recruited. Obviously when the larger motor units containing the most and the largest muscle fibers are recruited the tension will increase more than when the _____ units are recruited.

small

---

173. The rate of discharge of the motor unit will also contribute to the total tension. The greater tension will occur with the _____ frequencies.

higher

64

174. The motor neuron pool consists of the cell bodies of all the neurons which innervate all the muscle fibers in a given muscle. By the activation of combinations of these muscle and nerve cells all different grades of muscle tension and speed of contraction can be developed.

Sherrington originally suggested that motor neurons were arranged according to functional groups (Henneman, 1980).

Henneman & Mendell (1981) have described the motor neuron pool as being arranged by cell size which, as you know, is also an arrangement by cell excitability.

In either reflex responses or voluntary responses, the small tonic motor neurons tend to be activated before the large phasic ones. According to these researchers, it is apparent that the rank order of recruitment in the motor neuron pool could be rather strictly defined.

Generally, no matter what kind of output is desired, the order by which neurons are activated may be rather _____.

rigid

---

175. You may recall the discussion concerning the critical firing level of a neuron. No matter how the neuron is activated, it will discharge at the same point in relation to all the other motor neurons in the pool

Basmajian performed many well-known experiments with single motor unit control. With an EMG machine to provide visual and auditory feedback, most people can be trained to produce so minute a contraction that only one motor unit is activated in the area surveyed by the electrode used. An increase in tension first results from an increase in the frequency of the motor unit action potential. Any further increase in tension will then require recruitment of a second _____ _____.

motor unit

176. The first motor unit to be activated is always a small tonic unit. The second unit is larger. According to Henneman (1980) and others (Dietz & Young, 1984), no evidence has been shown that individuals clearly have true voluntary or conscious control over the **order** of recruitment.

It is not possible usually to recruit the larger motor units _____.

first

---

177. Experiments were also done in which the speed of muscle contractions were increased. During these increasingly faster contractions the motor neurons would be activated at a lower force level of muscle contraction than ordinarily happens during a slow contraction.

In other words, motor units of all sizes are synchronously recruited (Dietz & Young, 1984). That is, the high threshold units started firing sooner but they were not activated before the lower threshold units.

Complex muscles in which different parts of the muscle function in different ways during different movements show a somewhat different ability. Units can be activated in one part of the muscle by a particular movement and in another part of the muscle with a different movement without regard to the fine points of their size (Dietz & Young, 1984).

Recruitment based on the size principle may be most valid for muscles in which fibers insert on one long tendon. It may be less valid for more _____ muscles.

complex

---

178. In simple muscles, at least, the smallest neurons are activated _____.

first

179. Experiments with extremely rapid or bursting movements show that these movements are too fast to be controlled by sensory feedback from activated muscles. It is apparent that these movements are pre-programmed at the spinal level or must be sent to the motor neuron pool at the segmental level before the movement occurs.

The integration of pre-programmed activity is probably accomplished by pyramidal tract signals to the motor neurons. The point is, however, that even in such movements the large rapidly contracting motor units were not preferentially recruited.

During all types of movement it is likely that the first neurons to be recruited are the _____ ones.

small

180. Even the pre-programmed circuitry for certain movements appears to include recruitment of neurons according to the principle of their _____.

size

181. Recruitment of motor neurons appears to follow a rather rigid _____.

order

182. Many movements, particularly rapid or bursting movements, are most likely _____ at the spinal level.

pre-programmed

183. If you consider a motor neuron pool to be schematically drawn in a series according to size, (see following diagram) you can see that on the left are the small neurons which are most susceptible to activation. They differ relatively little in size from one another and there are many of them.

On the right are the large high threshold neurons which vary greatly in size and there are fewer of them.

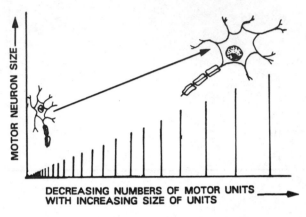

You can see that the smallest amount of force that can be added to that which is already present gets larger as the force of the contraction increases. Therefore, there is less fine control of tension if the tension which is present is very _____.

high

---

184. Do not forget that there are variations in contractile properties of the muscle units which are innervated by these motor neurons.

This variation helps to ensure the optimum function of the whole system for a wide variety of forces, loads, and speeds.

As tension requirements increase there is less _____ control of tension.

fine

185. We used to believe that the CNS could pick and choose from a wide variety of motor units to achieve a given movement. That is, if the pool contained 300 units, the CNS might use the units in many different combinations to achieve the desired total outputs.

The possible combination of active units in a pool of 300 would be on the order of 10^{90}. Selective activation, then, would require tremendous circuitry and an eternity of time for the necessary calculation to be accomplished (Henneman, 1980).

It would appear that a pool of cells which is activated by a simple rule in which the cells are recruited by size decreases the demand on the _CNS_.

CNS

---

186. Generally, in any activity, motor units will most likely be recruited in a pattern according to size. A small tonic motor neuron may be recruited first in **any** activity.

Does the CNS mobilize just the large, phasic and powerful motor units for the speed and power required in a high jump?

Answer: _No_

No, the smaller (or at least some of the smallest) units are recruited first.

---

187. Some evidence suggests that motor units may not be recruited solely by size. These are units which are found in _complex_ muscles.

complex

188. There have been other studies which have complicated the picture. Some have shown an apparent independent control of some fast twitch units. It has also been demonstrated that certain pathology can result in reversals of recruitment.

Some debate continues, therefore, as to how recruitment and purposeful movement are related. More than likely, however, the principle of motor neuron recruitment by size will remain a most significant, if not the total answer (Henneman, 1980; Bishop, 1982).

Remember also that is is likely that different motor neuron types exist even though they might be the same size. This, too, might account for a variety of _____ responses.

motor or recruitment

Under most conditions studied the large motor units appear to be recruited _____.

last

Some studies have shown that the order of recruitment is not completely _____.

fixed or rigid

In some investigations there was evidence of reversals in _____.

recruitment

_____

189. A study of the recruitment of fast and slow motor units during tonic and phasic contractions in **man** is basically in agreement with the size principle of recruitment (Maton, 1980).

It was shown that the same motor unit **may** discharge in both tonic and phasic contractions.

This observation is in agreement with the proposed recruitment based on the _____ principle.

size

190. This experiment also showed that in both tonic and phasic work the firing rate and recruitment depended only upon the external force it was working against.

For example, a particular motor unit which was not recruited for a low level tonic activity and which was recruited for a phasic activity could also be recruited in a tonic activity which was performed against a greater load (Maton, 1980).

The conclusion made by these investigators was that "tonic" and "phasic" characterize the motor unit twitches, but do not imply tonic-phasic functional differentiation.

The same motor unit can play a role in the gradation of both _tonic_ and _phasic_ contractions.

tonic
phasic

NOTE: The concept of functional differentiation is expanded by the work of Tokizane and Shimazu (1964). See pages 75 to 82.

191. You will recall that muscle is among the most plastic and mutable tissues. Muscle changes dramatically with the demand placed upon it.

The firing patterns of the neurons are thought to determine the contractile properties of muscle cells. The firing patterns of each type of motor neuron most likely differ sufficiently to explain the considerable variation in the contractile properties of muscle. It is possible, however, that differences other than the firing pattern influence muscle fibers.

It is important to remember that all muscle fibers in a _____ _____ are homogeneous.

muscle unit
or
motor unit

---

192. If a particular muscle has a greater percentage of one muscle fiber type than another, a muscle fiber type predominance is said to exist. When many individuals are examined and the information pooled the proportion of slow twitch to fast twitch fiber types is about 50:50. There is much variability, however, from person to person or from muscle to muscle within the same person.

If the vastus medialis has 80 percent slow twitch fibers it is said that there is a slow-twitch fiber _____.

predominance

---

193. All the muscle fibers in a motor unit are homogenous. All the muscle fibers in a **muscle** are not of the same type.

The predominance of muscle fiber types both among inidividuals and different muscles in the same individual is quite _____.

variable

72

194. Muscle biopsies of world class athletes have opened many avenues of discovery and speculation concerning muscle mutability. Muscle biopses of the gastrocnemius muscles of world class runners show a definite composition that is most suited to each of the athlete's particular events.

In sprinters, 60 percent of the fibers were type II; in middle distance runners 40-60 percent of the fibers were type I and in endurance runners more than 60 percent were type I fibers. Conversely, in world class weight lifters as many as 83 percent of the muscle fibers were type II (McCafferty & Horvath, 1977).

Studies with other types of athletes have not always shown such a clear predominance pattern. Evaluating the literature is also difficult because the muscles most accessible for testing may not be those most functionally active in the movement.

Nonetheless, evidence would point to the possibility that performance in some activities is directly related to the fiber-type predominance in certain _m_.

muscles

---

195. In certain muscles at least, world class endurance runners have a predominance of type _____ muscle fibers.

I(SO)

---

196. Sprinters may have a predominance of type _____ muscle fibers.

II(FOG & FG)

197. Investigators have also confirmed the differentiation of motor units through physiological studies on normal humans (Tokizane & Shimazu, 1964). These studies were performed through EMG recordings of single motor units during the physiologic activity of active muscle contraction.

These investigators recorded the intervals between the activation and re-activation of the motor unit during contraction.

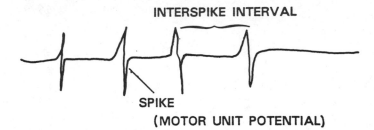

INTERSPIKE INTERVAL

SPIKE
(MOTOR UNIT POTENTIAL)

Generally speaking, a weak contraction results from a low frequency discharge (long inter-spike intervals) and strong contractions result from _____ frequency discharges (short inter-spike _____).

high
intervals

---

198. Close inspection of the spike to spike intervals show certain irregularities that cannot be changed no matter how hard the individual tries to keep the muscle contraction constant.

During strong contractions the intervals are short and relatively regular. During weak contractions the intervals are longer and more irregular.

Regularity of the inter-spike intervals depends, in part, upon the strength of the muscle _____.

contraction

199. Obviously, the inter-spike interval will be smaller in conditions of _____high_____ frequency discharge.

high

---

200. The inter-spike interval is also more regular in _____Strong_____ contractions.

strong

---

201. The investigators plotted the duration of inter-spike intervals from the motor unit with decreasing levels of contraction:

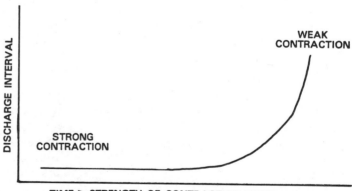

MODIFIED FROM TOKIZANE AND SHIMAZU: FUNCTIONAL DIFFERENTIATION OF HUMAN SKELETAL MUSCLE--CORTILIZATION AND SPINALIZATION OF MOVEMENT. CHARLES THOMAS, SPRINGFIELD, IL., 1964

This graph shows that the discharge intervals are short when the motor unit is performing a strong contraction, and that the intervals are long when performing a _____weak_____ contraction.

weak

202. The graph also shows that there is a period when the intervals are similar (plateau) and a point at which the curve rapidly rises.

The curve rises most sharply when the contractions are _____.

weaker

---

203. Plots of the duration of inter-spike intervals were done for many motor units in a particular muscle. When this was done the combined intervals cluster along two definite curves.

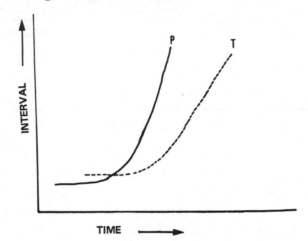

MODIFIED FROM TOKIZANE AND SHIMAZU: FUNCTIONAL DIFFERENTIATION OF HUMAN SKELETAL MUSCLE--CORTILIZATION AND SPINALIZATION OF MOVEMENT. CHARLES THOMAS, SPRINGFIELD, IL., 1964

For the soleus muscle the units involved in the P-curve maintain a constant rhythmiticity of discharge at the highest frequencies of about 33 per second to 15 per second. Then the curve turns upward, showing that as the contraction becomes weaker the rate of discharge becomes irregular.

The P-curve would most likely represent the most phasic type of _____ unit.

motor

NOTE: Tokizane and Shimazu actually called this curve the K-curve for "Kinetic" motor units. It should be less confusing to call it a P-curve for "phasic" motor units. In the interest of clarity, we have taken that liberty.

204. The T-curve has a much longer plateau than the P-curve. The discharge intervals do not become as rapidly irregular when the discharge rate is slowed and the contraction gets weaker.

The T-units show a regular pattern down to about 8 repetitions per second. In other words, the T-unit muscle fibers are most suitable for a smooth and steady contraction.

The T-curve would most likely represent the ___*tonic*___ type of motor unit.

tonic

---

205. Based on this inter-spike interval information, Tokizane and Shimazu (1964) concluded that there are two functionally different kinds of motor units. They found both kinds of units in essentially all the different muscles they examined.

Investigators utilizing exclusively physiological data recorded from humans have also concluded that motor units can be classified into two general categories: ___*tonic*___ and ___*phasic*___.

tonic (I)
phasic (II)

---

206. These same researchers also found that phasic and tonic motor units were distributed in a particular pattern within muscles.

Tonic motor units were more commonly found near the central axis of the muscle. The phasic motor units were distributed away from the central axis of the muscle.

It would appear that the different motor unit types are specifically located within certain areas of the _____.

muscle

207. The next step in these experiments was to compare the P-curves and T-curves in different muscles. These observations revealed some striking features of the organization of human musculature (Tokizane & Shimazu, 1964).

Muscles of the upper extremity showed the same curves as those of the soleus, but they were shifted to the left. That is, muscles of the upper extremity are more phasic than those of the lower extremity.

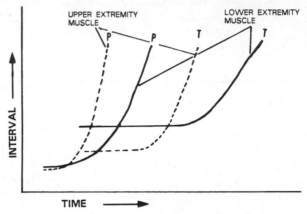

MODIFIED FROM TOKIZANE AND SHIMAZU: FUNCTIONAL DIFFERENTIATION OF HUMAN SKELETAL MUSCLE--CORTILIZATION AND SPINALIZATION OF MOVEMENT.

As you might expect, muscles of the forearm are more phasic than those of the upper _____.

arm

---

208. The facial muscles are the most phasic of all muscles. The obicularis oculi, in fact, had no T-curve at all.

Based on this information, we would expect these muscles to discharge at a very high rate. In fact, steady activity at low frequencies such as 8 or 10 spikes per second is very difficult with tongue and eye muscles (Tokizane & Shimazu, 1964).

The anal sphincter, on the other hand, has tonic motor units which discharge as low as 3 spikes per second, and this contraction is maintained constantly.

The anal sphincter would be an example of a muscle composed of many _____ units.

tonic

78

209. A graph was done of two muscles in the hand and foot which are homologs. The abductor pollicis brevis and abductor hallucis showed distinct differences: the motor units of the hand muscle were shifted much more to the left (phasic) than those of the foot muscle.

It could be concluded that the muscles behave differently depending on whether they are located in the upper or lower extremity.

It can be seen that the motor units have a wide variation in _phasic_ and _tonic_ characteristics.

phasic
tonic

---

210. The tonic motor unit of a facial muscle is more phasic than the phasic motor unit of the anal muscle (Tokizane & Shimazu, 1964).

This data would tell us that there is a wide variation in the functional characteristics of motor units. It is difficult to account for the intermediate or type IIA motor unit in these observations. It would be logical to assume that these are the units which fall between the two curves.

The more tonic nature of the motor units in muscles of the foot compared to the hand would seem quite suited to the function of the foot muscles as _tonic_ muscles.

postural
or
tonic

---

211. Tokizane and Shimazu noted that while the soleus cooperates with the gastrocnemius in maintaining the standing posture, the soleus is more tonic in nature than the gastrocnemius.

The tibialis anterior shows more phasic motor units in the superficial layer of the muscle and the deeper layers have more _____ units.

tonic

79

212. The superficial muscles of the back (latissimus dorsi and longissimus) are phasic in nature. The deeper multifidus muscle is predominantly _____.

tonic

---

213. In the abdominal musculature, the superficial rectus femoris is more phasic, while the tonic internal oblique is a _____ muscle.

deeper

---

214. Studies in which the inter-spike interval in motor units have been recorded in man under the physiologic conditions of normal muscle contraction compliment those which involve the histochemical analysis of muscle tissue biopsies.

The former studies show the differentiation into tonic and phasic (I and II) motor units, but most importantly they show the wide variety of functional differentiation among muscles.

Pictured below is a composite graph of many muscles. The solid lines are the P-curves and the broken lines represent the T-curves:

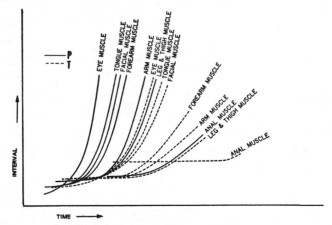

MODIFIED FROM TOKIZANE AND SHIMAZU: FUNCTIONAL DIFFERENTIATION OF HUMAN SKELETAL MUSCLE--CORTILIZATION AND SPINALIZATION OF MOVEMENT.

This diagram shows that the tonic motor units of the most phasic muscles are still more phasic than the phasic motor units of the _____ muscles.

tonic

80

215. Fill in the following chart:

Phasic	Tonic
gastrocnemius	_Soleus_
ant. tibialis (superficial)	_deep ant. tibialis_
longissimus	_multifidis_
rectus abdominus	_obliques_
forearm muscles	_upper arm ms._
abductor pollicis	_abductor hallicus_
15-30 contractions/sec	_3-15/second_

soleus
ant. tibialis (deep)
multifidis
obliques
upper arm muscles
abductor hallucis
3-15/second

---

216. Muscle fiber-type differences vary from muscle to muscle in the same individual and from individual to individual as well. Some experimental data show that even within types there is a wide variation of functional differentiation.

Some type I units appear to be more tonic than other ___type I___ units.

type I

NOTE: The strict bimodal distribution found by Tokizane & Shimazu has not been substantiated. That is, most investigators find a large population of intermediate fibers as well. We have already noted this condition. The information as presented is useful for conceptualization of the extremes in the motor unit population.

The observations that different muscles exhibit different ranges of steady firing rates has indeed been substantiated. The more tonic nature of the proximal muscles and the caudal musculature appears to be quite valid (Burke, 1981).

81

217. Weight lifters, at least world class weight lifters, may have a predominance of type _____ muscle fibers.

II(FOG & FG)

---

218. It stands to reason that if sprinting and weight lifting do not depend on oxygen consumption and activities such as long distance running do, long distance athletes would rely more heavily on type _____ muscle fibers.

I(SO)

---

219. These patterns of predominance would seem logical if you consider the requirements for performing these athletic endeavors at a world class level.

The question then arises: if we could change an individual's muscle fiber composition, could we perhaps engineer athletic prowess?

Animal studies have shown that muscle fiber types can be changed through at least three mechanisms.

If the muscle fibers are cross-innervated, that is, a type I fiber is matched to a type II neuron and vice versa the muscle fibers will, indeed, change to match their new innervation (Eccles and Buller, 1960).

Type I muscle fibers innervated by type II motor neurons will become type _____ fibers.

II

---

220. It also appears that some type I motor units such as those in the face are more phasic than some type II motor units such as those in the _____ sphincter (Tokizane & Shimazu, 1964).

anal

221. It has been shown that a chronic constant low frequency electrical stimulation for 24 hours a day to type II muscle fibers for a period of months will change them to type I (Pette, 1976; Vrbova, 1979).

Type II fibers can be changed to type I fibers by _elec._ _Stim_.

electrical stimulation

---

222. Animal experiments involving weight lifting exercises have also shown some influences in changing fiber types, particularly in the young animal (Jaweed, et.al., 1977).

So it appears that fiber types can be altered, but the successful research protocols used in animal studies are usually not acceptable in human experimentation. Some changes have been noted with electrical stimulation protocols (Munsat, 1976).

The literature is replete with attempts to alter the muscle fiber composition in humans through various types of exercises. These have not met with much success.

Because of such failures it has been suggested that an individual's muscle fiber composition is genetically determined. In this case, world class athletes could be said to be born for their particular _sport_.

sport

---

223. Some investigations in which endurance versus strength exercises were studied in humans seem to indicate that the type II fibers may have the capability of shifting within their sub-groups (Anderson, 1977).

That is, an endurance exercise regimen may cause a shift in the composition of type II fibers from IIB to _IIA_.

IIA

83

224. Tokizane and Shimazu (1964) also studied the possibility of altering motor unit types with activity. They examined the inter-spike intervals from motor units of the rectus femoris muscles of three stevedores. These men perform jobs which require carrying of heavy loads on the shoulders.

When comparing the P-curves and T-curves of these stevedores versus untrained individuals, the difference was striking.

There was a marked shift of the T-curve to the right and some rightward shift of the P-curve as well. That is, the units became more tonic over time. This was most remarkable in a man of 25 years of service and less so with one of 20 years of service. The smallest shift was with a stevedore of 12 years of service.

This study shows the possibility of fiber type change under stress. If it actually represents change of fiber types, the most noticeable element is the length of time necessary to produce these changes.

It would not be hard to understand why no changes were noted in subjects who exercised a few times a week for a few weeks.

Change of muscle fiber types in man may require consistent exercise for a _____ _____.

long time

---

225. A strength protocol may result in a shift of type IIA to a greater number of _____ fibers.

IIB

---

226. It is also apparent that even though one fiber type does not completely shift to another fiber type with activity, it may become more "tonic" or "phasic" than it was before _____.

exercise

227. Thus, it appears that shifts between type I and type II muscle fibers probably do not occur in humans under normal exercise conditions.

It may be possible in humans, however, to create shifts in fiber predominance between type _IIA_ and _IIB_ .

IIA
IIB

---

228. It is also possible that shifts in muscle fiber type would be evident if an activity is performed daily for _years_ .

years

---

229. Undoubtedly, exercise "fine tunes" the system. Additional contractile proteins are synthesized and the muscle fibers hypertrophy. The anaerobic and aerobic capacities are enhanced. Thus, the muscle responds to the demands placed upon it whatever the composition.

It may also be possible to cause a shift in the sub-groups of type _II_ fibers.

II

---

230. It may not be possible to change muscle fibers from type I to type II or vice versa with exercise. It would be beneficial, however, to exercise muscles with desired functional activities in mind.

Specific exercise should enhance the _____ and _____ capacities of the muscle.

anaerobic
aerobic

231. Recent evidence has shown that muscle fibers may "split" longitudinally after reaching a certain size, thus, contributing to changes in cross-sectional area and fiber type predominance.

There is a large body of literature concerning muscle fiber types and their alterations which will not be presented here.

The point of this brief review is that muscle which undergoes training activities does respond to the _____ placed upon it.

demands

---

232. We know that muscles have a variable predominance of muscle fiber types which differs among muscles in the same individuals and among different individuals.

It could also be theorized that an individual with a lower proportion of type I muscle fibers might fatigue more rapidly during endurance activities. This could result in joint or soft tissue injury by failure to protect the joints from exercise loading (Rose & Rothstein, 1982).

Fiber type predominance may, therefore, be a factor in a predisposition to _____ or _____ _____ injury.

joint
soft tissue

---

233. Conversely, an individual with a type I fiber predominance may not be able to generate tension rapidly in response to sudden loads (Rose & Rothstein, 1982).

This also could result in _____
_____.

joint or soft
tissue injury

234. Studies on normal athletes have led to questions concerning the relationship of disease states to particular muscle fiber types. These types of studies are proliferating and will undoubtedly continue to contribute to and change our understanding of muscle alterations in many different diseases and disorders.

Let us consider some of the research findings relative to muscle fiber types and disease. As you might expect, there are numerous types of derangements within muscle fibers with disease states. These may include shape changes, enzyme abnormalities, atrophic and hypertrophic muscle cells, changes in membrane structure and changes in the many organelles themselves. We will not consider all these changes in detail. What is important is that you get a general idea of the selectivity of fiber type changes.

For example, in disuse atrophy there is selective atrophy of type II fibers. The greatest difficulty would then be loss in overall "strength" or the ability to generate peak tension _rapidly_.

rapidly

---

235. In the muscular dystrophies there are usually hypertrophic muscle cells and a deficiency in certain fiber types. In Duchenine muscular dystrophy and in myotonia congenita, for example, there is a deficiency in type IIB fibers.

In disuse atrophy there is also selective atrophy of type _II_ fibers.

II

---

236. An inability to generate adequate tension rapidly could indicate that the individual has selectively lost type _II_ fibers.

II

237. Some of the problems such as disuse atrophy are self-limiting and completely or near completely reversible. Others are progressive in nature. These factors should be taken into consideration in rehabilitation planning. It is possible that even the most progressive disorder may be altered postively and this fact should not be ignored in the treatment plan.

The treatment of selective atrophy may require the inclusion of selective _____.

exercise

---

238. With denervation all fiber types are involved. Fiber "grouping" occurs. If there is reinnervation, the intact nearby motor units may send out "collateral sprouts" and reinnervate the denervated fibers. These reinnervated fibers are changed to the type of the surviving motor neuron and thus a larger area appears homogenous. This is referred to as "grouping."

If a type II motor unit innervates a type I muscle fiber, the muscle fiber will become a _____ _____ fiber.

type II

---

239. In some muscular dystrophies there is a deficiency of type _____ fibers.

IIB

---

240. "Grouping" occurs when there is reinnervation of denervated muscle cells by nearby motor units which send out _____ _____.

collateral sprouts

241. Type IIA or IIB atrophy may be found in patients with CVA, those on corticosteroid therapy and in myasthenia gravis. In fact, type II atrophy has been described in almost all serious chronic debilitating diseases (Rose and Rothstein, 1982).

With some or all of these conditions, the therapist may wish to consider exercises which may most likely recruit and stimulate these fibers. A word of caution -- effective training of type II fibers requires maximal efforts in tension or speed. This would have to be monitored carefully and would perhaps b' unwise in some patients.

The point is, diseases do not have to be diseases of muscle, or even of the motor unit, to cause actual selective structural and functional changes 'n *muscle*

muscle

---

242. Knowledge of muscle physiology and pathophysiology should be prerequisite to the treatment of **any** type of patient because invariably there is likely to be some alteration in the *muscle* itself.

muscle

---

243. It is not the intent of the authors to present suggested treatment for specific diseases and disorders. The most important point is that physical therapists should be the most knowledgeable of professionals relative to muscle physiology and pathophysiology. If the changes and conditions of many or most diseases also result in changes in muscle, it is logical that muscle would respond to treatment.

Some of the most effective results in the clinic will undoubtedly be from alterations in musculo-skeletal alignment, in balance, and in _____ tissue itself.

muscle

SUMMARY

The motor unit is the smallest functional component of the neuromuscular system. It consists of the: (1) motor neuron which includes (a) the cell body and (b) its axon and terminal branches; (2) the neuromuscular junctions; and (3) all the muscle fibers which that neuron innervates.

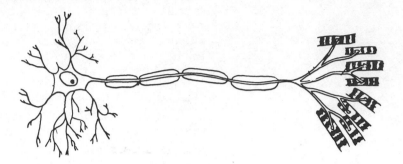

This peripheral motor system is the final common pathway for the expression of sensory input. Nervous system activity converges on this final pathway to produce or prevent a single event--muscle contraction. When the motor neuron cell body is excited to the threshold level the entire motor unit responds in an "all-or-nothing" mode.

MOTOR UNIT TYPE

	I	IIA	IIB
Motor neuron cell size	small	intermediate	large
Critical firing level	earliest	intermediate	latest
Susceptibility to inhibition	least	intermediate	greatest
Susceptibility to post-tetanic potentiation	greatest	intermediate	least
Duration of hyperpolarization after-potentials	longest	intermediate	shortest
Axons			
cross-sectional area	smallest	intermediate	largest
conduction velocity	slowest	intermediate	fastest
NMJ Type	I	IIA	IIB
Susceptibility to PTP	greatest	intermediate	least
Muscle fibers			
size	smallest	intermediate	largest
fatiguability	least	intermediate	most
speed of contraction	slowest	intermediate	fastest
maximal tension	lowest	intermediate	highest
oxygen system	yes	yes	no
glycolytic	no	yes	yes
Consequence of activity	slow, gross, posture movements	fast	rapid, precise phasic movement

There is often confusion surrounding the labels given to the motor neuron. The motor neuron may be referred to as the anterior horn cell. Often the term "motor neuron" is used to refer to the cell body. To eliminate confusion the term is defined as follows:

> **Motor neuron** (anterior horn cell; alpha motor neuron)--the entire nerve cell including the cell body and its processes.

The total tension a given muscle can generate is determined in large part by: (1) the total number of muscle fibers activated; and (2) the total tension produced by each mucle fiber.

Motor units may be somewhat classified as **phasic** or **tonic,** and all of the muscle fibers in one motor unit are homogenous.

Motor units which contain many muscle fibers and are particularly activated when great levels of tension are required. Motor units with very few muscle fibers are responsible for fine, controlled movements.

The total tension which a muscle develops depends upon the total number of motor units recruited and the size of the motor units recruited. Greater tension will also occur with greater discharge frequencies of the motor units.

Recent investigators (Henneman, 1980) have postulated that the order of recruitment of motor neurons occurs according to the size of the motor neurons. This is called the **Size Principle** of recruitment. The small tonic motor neurons tend to be activated first in either voluntary or reflex responses. When the speed of muscle contractions increase all units come in earlier but remain in the same order.

Studies on humans have shown that the same motor units may discharge in both tonic and phasic contractions. This data supports the size principle of motor neuron recruitment.

Muscle is among the most plastic of tissues and muscle changes dramatically with the demand placed upon it. Many studies involve the adaptation of muscle length to lengthened and shortened positions. These are not elaborated upon in this text.

If a particular muscle has a greater percentage of one muscle fiber type than another, a muscle fiber type predominance is said to exist. Muscle biopsies of the gastrocnemius muscles of some world class runners show that sprinters have 60 percent type II fibers, middle distance runners have 40-60 percent type II fibers, and endurance runners have less than 40 percent. Evidence would point to the possibility that performance in some activities is directly related to fiber type predominance in certain muscles.

Experiments in which the duration of inter-spike intervals were measured in EMG recording from contracting muscles support the differentiation of motor units into two groups: phasic (type II) and tonic (type I). These experiments show some other interesting differentiations:

(1) Tonic motor units are found nearer the central axis of the muscle than phasic ones are.

(2) Deep portions of the muscle contain more tonic motor units; superficial portions more phasic ones.

(3)   Muscles have the following order relative to the most phasic to the most tonic: eye, face, tongue, hand, forearm and arm. The upper extremities are more phasic than the lower extremities.

(4)   Homologs in the hands and feet (abductor pollicis and abductor hallucis) are completely different. The foot muscle is clearly more tonic than the hand muscle.

(5)   Complimentary muscles (synergists) have different compositions:
-the soleus is more tonic than the gastrocnemius
-the deep back and abdominal muscles (multifidus and obliques) are more tonic than the lateral and superficial ones (longissimus and rectus abdominus)

The evidence shows that some type I units are more tonic than other type I units. That is, some are suited to function smoothly at very low frequencies while others require that the frequency be a little higher for optimum function. The same observation holds true for phasic or type II motor units.

Tokizane (1964) showed distinct shifts in T-curves (tonic) to the right in stevedores of 12-25 years of service. The findings were greater as the years of service in this strenuous endeavor increased. Recent studies with athletes fail to show clear fiber type shifts, although some shifting may occur between the sub-types of the phasic motor units: type IIA and IIB. It is possible that findings are not more dramatic because the intensity and duration of the exercise regimens are not sufficient enough to effect a clear change.

Fiber type predominance may be a factor in predisposition to joint and soft tissue injury.

Changes in muscle are fiber type specific in certain disease states. Selective atrophy and hypertrophy occurs in many chronic diseases such as muscular dystrophy, disuse, denervation, CVA, cerebral palsy and so forth. Diseases do not have to be of the muscle to cause selective structural and functional changes.

Knowledge of muscle physiology and pathophysiology should be prerequisite to the treatment of **any** type of patient because invariably there is likely to be some alteration in the muscle itself.

SECTION II

The Muscle Spindle

1. Sensory Receptors

2. Types of Receptors

3. Classification of Nerve Fiber Types

4. Muscle Receptors

   a. The Muscle Spindle
      1. The Primary Afferent Receptor
      2. The Secondary Receptor

   b. The Golgi Tendon Organ

5. Interneurons

6. The Motor or Efferent System to the Muscle Spindle

7. Control of Alpha and Gamma Neurons

SENSORY RECEPTORS

1. Before looking at specific peripheral sensory receptors, it should be useful to review some of the principles of sensory processing. It is clear that the nervous system functions on electrical energy. Yet the sensations or information in the external world that the CNS needs to know about come in many energy forms. Vision relates to light waves, touch to mechanical energy, taste to chemical energy, and so forth. How do these different energy forms become known to the CNS?

   Sensory input begins with a receptor. The function of a receptor is to behave as a transducer. A transducer transforms one kind of energy into another.

   A sensory receptor functions as a _transducer_ of energy forms.

transducer

---

2. The Pacinian corpuscle, a pressure receptor, will serve as an example. The corpuscle consists of a number of concentric lamellae composed of connective tissue. The receptor itself is the peripheral end of the sensory nerve fiber which is surrounded by the lamellar capsule.

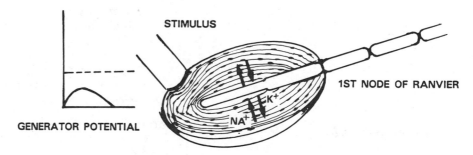

STIMULUS

1ST NODE OF RANVIER

K⁺

NA⁺

GENERATOR POTENTIAL

   When pressure is applied to the capsule it is deformed and the mechanical energy is carried to the axon terminal. A local change in membrane potential of the terminal occurs. This is called a generator potential.

   A generator potential is a _local_ change in membrane potential.

local

95

3. A stimulus will result in a generator potential of a particular amplitude. If the stimulus is increased in intensity the amplitude will also _____.

increase

THRESHOLD - - - - - -

GENERATOR POTENTIAL

4. As the intensity increases the amplitude of the generator potential increases. Put another way, we can say that the generator potential amplitude varies through a wide range of responses. There is never any refractory period of hyperpolarization. The generator response obviously does not follow the all-or-none law of activation.

The amplitude can change with differences in stimulus _____.

intensity

5. When the amplitude is great enough to reach the threshold value for the first node of Ranvier an action potential is generated along the axon into the spinal cord. The action potential follows the all-or-none law.

The generator potential is a non-propagated current, the action potential is a _____ current.

propagated

ACTION POTENTIAL

THRESHOLD - - - -

NA⁺ K⁺

6. The generator potential does not leave the area of the receptor. The action potential, however, is propagated along the *axon* .

axon

---

7. Generator potentials can be summed. That is, inputs which come from different places on the receptor or which result from rapid repetitive impulses will alter the amplitude of the *generator potential* .

generator potential

---

8. The amplitude of the generator potential may be summed and graded through a wide range of responses. The amplitude of the action potential is fixed.

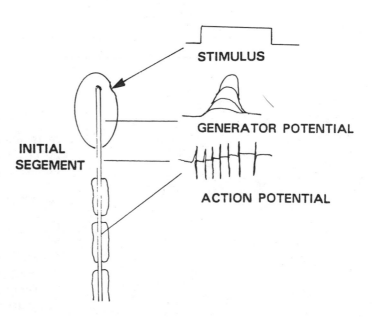

Action potentials, therefore, cannot be _____ or _____ .

graded
summed

9. An action potential is an "all-or-none" phenomenon. Either a threshold is reached and an action potential is generated or nothing happens.

    In order to generate an action potential the membrane at the initial segment must reach a _____ value.

threshold

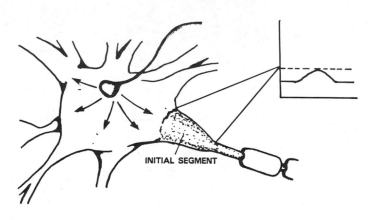

INITIAL SEGMENT

---

10. It is apparent that generator potentials and action potentials have opposite characteristics. Fill in the blanks on the chart.

Generator Potentials	Action Potentials
1. variable amplitude	_____
2. _____	cannot be summed
3. non-propagated	_____
4. confined to the receptor area	_____
5. graded responses	_____

1. fixed amplitude
2. summed
3. propagated
4. moving, not confined
5. all-or-none

98

11. If the action potential has a fixed amplitude how does the CNS receive information about the **intensity** of the stimulus? Stimulus intensity is coded by the frequency of the action potential. A large amplitude generator potential will cause repetitive depolarization of the axon.

The larger the amplitude of the generator potential the greater the frequency of the *action* potential.

action

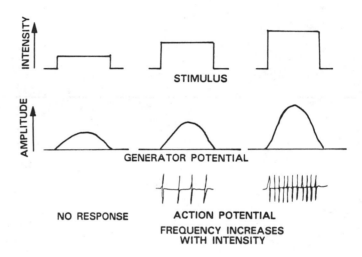

NO RESPONSE   ACTION POTENTIAL
FREQUENCY INCREASES
WITH INTENSITY

12. Sensory information is transduced into electrical energy through the process by which the receptor produces a _____ _____.

generator potential

13. The generator potential has many properties in common with the excitatory post synaptic potentials of nerve cells and the end plate potentials of the neuromuscular _____.

junction

99

14. The generator potential transforms energy impinging upon the receptor into electrical energy--the action potential. The action potential carries the information into the _____.

CNS

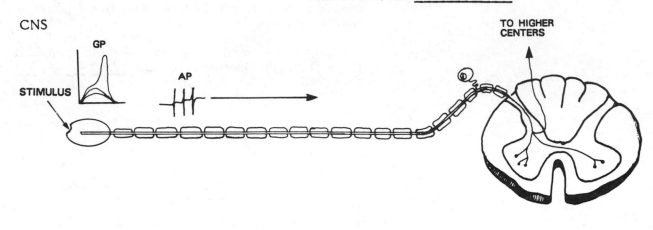

15. Action potentials cannot be _____ or _____.

graded
summed

16. An increasing intensity of the stimulus is coded in the CNS by increasing the _____ of the action potential.

frequency

17. The area of the afferent nerve cell which must reach threshold for an action potential to be generated is the _____ _____.

initial segment

TYPES OF RECEPTORS

18. Receptors generally fall into two functional categories: those that are rapidly adapting and those that are _____ adapting.

slowly

---

19. The rapidly adapting receptor produces a discharge when the stimulus is applied and then the generator potential amplitude drops off even though the stimulus is still present.

STIMULUS

RAPIDLY ADAPTING RECEPTOR

ON   OFF

The receptor may then produce another series of potentials after the stimulus is _____.

removed

---

20. A rapidly adapting receptor may produce a response only when the stimulus is _____ and _____.

applied
removed

21. Slowly adapting receptors respond to long lasting stimluli with persisting generator responses. These potentials elicit repetitive action potentials in their axons.

Just as with the rapidly adapting receptor, there are augmented bursts of activity when the stimulus is applied and removed ("on" and "off" responses), however, there is also persistent output as long as the stimulus is _____.

maintained

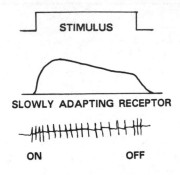

22. With non-adapting or slowly adapting receptors, there is a persistent output during a maintained stimulus. The rate or frequency of discharge is essentially in linear relationship with the stimulus intensity, although there is usually a steady decline in output as the stimulus is maintained.

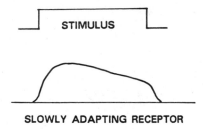

From a functional perspective, it is nice that certain kinds of stimuli are not constantly bombarding our awareness. Consider how harried you would be by the end of the day if you were constantly aware of your clothes, the room temperature and so forth.

The receptor responsiveness decreases or the generator potential fails to produce action potentials at some point after the stimulus is applied to a _____ _____ receptor.

rapidly adapting

23. On the other hand, we need relatively constant feedback from some receptors which tell us about our movements, positions and environment.

   Action potentials continue to be generated during a maintained stimulus in a _____ _____ receptor.

slowly adapting

---

24. It was stated earlier that the amplitude of the action potential is fixed and, therefore, intensity is coded in the nervous system by the _____ of action potentials.

frequency

---

25. From a treatment perspective, it is useful to know whether a receptor you wish to activate is rapidly or slowly adapting.

   To be of therapeutic value the former would require repetitive input and the latter would require only that the stimulus be _____.

maintained

---

26. The intensity and quality of the response to stimuli are also coded into the nervous system by mechanisms other than action potential frequency. Two examples of other coding mechanisms are the pattern of activation of different receptors and the number of receptors which are activated.

   Various mechamisms may be utilized by the nervous system for coding _____ information.

sensory

27. It has been fairly well established that each receptor is excited by a specific stimulus. This is termed modality specificity.

Knowledge and theories about receptors have come full circle. At one time anatomists believed that there was a specific type of receptor for every quality of sensation. Then physiologists suggested that sensory perception was only a matter of the pattern of activation of sensory receptors rather than a specific anatomic structure. Now we have come back to modality specificity, but some aspects of the pattern theory remain.

Perception of sensory input is a complex phenomenon involving CNS integration as well as the activation of specific receptors in various numbers and patterns.

The sensory endings of peripheral nerve fibers are differentially sensitive to one type of impinging _____.

energy, modality,
or sensation

---

28. Receptors can be generally classified as being _____ _____ or _____ _____.

rapidly adapting
slowly adapting

---

29. One mechanism by which sensory information is coded in the nervous system is by the _____ of _____ potentials.

frequency
action

---

30. A slowly adapting receptor can be activated during treatment when the stimulus is applied and _____.

maintained

31. As the stimulus strength becomes stronger the amplitudes of the _____ _____ increases.

generator potential

32. Most likely each receptor will respond to a _____ stimulus.

specific

33. If you wish to activate a rapidly adapting receptor during treatment, the stimulus will have to be _____.

repeated

34. A sensory receptor behaves as a _____.

transducer

35. When the amplitude of the generator potential reaches threshold an _____ _____ is generated.

action potential

36. Sensory nerve cells have axons as do anterior horn cells and all other types of nerve cells. Technically, by definition the long process which courses from the receptor to the dorsal root ganglion is called a dendrite (information is carried **to** the cell body). Except for transmitting in the opposite direction, these processes have all the same anatomical and physiological properties as the axons.

We will consider all these long processes whether they are part of sensory or motor cells to be _____.

axons

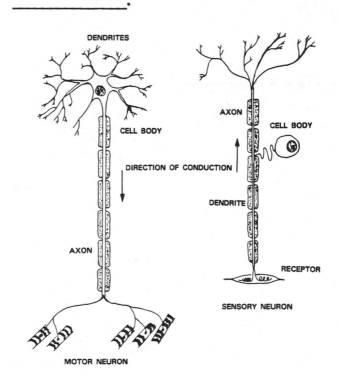

37. By definition, processes which carry information to the cell body are dendrites. Processes which carry information away from the cell body are axons.

Nonetheless, we will consider the long process which brings information from the periphery to the dorsal root ganglion to be an _____.

axon

38. You have perhaps wondered how some nerve fibers have received their names. For example, the axon serving the anterior horn cell body is called an **alpha** fiber. You will shortly encounter beta and gamma fibers, as well as A, B, and C fibers and I, II and III fibers and so forth. These names simply result from two classification systems which are based solely on the **size** of the axon.

   The Greek word **alpha** and, the letter A, are both the beginning of the alphabet and would logically represent the _____ largest/smallest axons.

largest

---

39. The Roman numeral I could also represent the _____ axons.

largest

---

40. These classifications were made by two different researchers, one was investigating dorsal root fibers and the other classified ventral root fibers. These fibers are all represented on the following chart.

Dorsal Root Fibers	Ventral Root Fibers	Conduction Velocities (a function of axon diameter)
I	A-alpha	75-120 m/sec
II	A-beta-gamma	35-75 m/sec
III	A-delta	5-30 m/sec
	B	3-15 m/sec
IV	C	.05-2 m/sec

   The smallest fibers which are lightly myelinated or unmyelinated are labeled IV or _____ fibers.

C

107

41. B fibers have unique properties and are pre-
ganglionic fibers of the autonomic nervous system.
They will not be included in further discussions in this
text.

There are no B type fibers in the _____
roots.

dorsal

---

42. A size fibers are subdivided into classes which are
identified by the Greek letters **alpha, beta, gamma**
and **delta.**

The fastest conducting A fibers are the A alpha
fibers. The slowest conducting fibers in the A class
are the _____.

A delta

---

43. Anterior horn cell bodies are served by the largest
and fastest fibers in the ventral root, the _____
fibers.

A alpha (or I)

---

44. In the literature, these dorsal and ventral root
classification systems are often equated and mixed.
Therefore, sensory fibers may be called A fibers even
though they were originally labeled with the Roman
numeral _____.

I

---

45. Fibers which are classified as I, II and III are also all
_____ fibers.

A

46. Sometimes the A-alpha system is abbreviated and fibers are simply referred to as alpha or beta or _____ fibers.

gamma
or
delta

---

47. There are other properties of these fibers that will be explored later. For the present, it is important to remove any mystery from such labels so that you know what an alpha or a gamma fiber is. Axons are classified according to their _____.

size

---

48. In this book, we are going to refer to all axons as A (alpha-delta), B or C fibers. Use of this system should help prevent confusion with muscle and joint receptors and motor units which are labeled with Roman numerals.

No matter whether the nerve fibers are sensory or motor in function, in this book they will be classified as _____, _____ and _____.

A
B
C

NOTE: The Roman numeral form will be cited parenthetically because you will encounter such terminology in the literature.

---

49. The classification of fibers into A-beta-gamma would suggest a range of sizes. The beta fibers would be the _____.

larger

beta-gamma

50. The dorsal root fibers labeled II correspond to the A _____ fibers.

51. The terms "A fiber" and "C fiber" as used in the literature may refer to either _____ or _____ fibers.

sensory (or dorsal root)
motor (or ventral root)

52. The slowest conducting fibers may be called either _____ or _____ fibers.

IV
C

53. The speed with which an action potential is conducted along the axon is determined by the _____ of the axon.

size

54. The alpha motor neuron is the equivalent in size to the fiber labeled with a Roman numeral _____.

I

SUMMARY

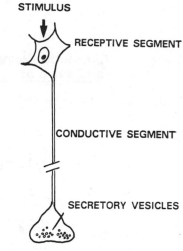

STIMULUS

RECEPTIVE SEGMENT

CONDUCTIVE SEGMENT

SECRETORY VESICLES

TRANSMISSIVE SEGMENT

A sensory nerve cell consists of (1) a specialized segment which is receptive to a specific stimulus, (2) an axon or conductive segment, and (3) a transmissive segment, the central terminus which contains the secretory vesicles.

Sensory receptors behave as transducers by reacting to one form of energy (such as mechanical energy) and triggering action potentials (electrical energy) in the axons. Thus, all forms of energy can be transduced or "translated" into electrical energy, the "language" of the nervous system.

One mechanism for the coding of stimulus intensity is through the frequency of action potentials conducted along the axon. The frequency of action potentials is determined by the amplitude of the generator potential which is directly related to the stimulus intensity.

Sensory receptors may be generally classified as rapidly adapting or slowly adapting. Clinically, the former would be stimulated through repetitive application of the stimulus. The latter would continue to respond as long as the stimulus is maintained.

Sensory receptors may also be classified as **exteroceptors** (external environment), **proprioceptors** (position) and **interoceptors** (internal environment). Within each of these categories will be both rapidly and slowly adapting receptors.

The conductive segments or axons of the sensory neurons may also be classified. This classification is according to cross-sectional area of the axon. The size of the axon determines the speed with which potentials may be conducted along the axon.

The fibers or axons have been labeled with both Roman numerals and Arabic letters with Greek subscripts. The same size fiber could be labeled II or A-gamma, depending upon its location, i.e. the dorsal or ventral roots.

Dorsal Root Fibers	Ventral Root Fibers	Conduction Velocities (a function of axon diameter)
I	A-alpha	75-120 m/sec
II	A-beta-gamma	35-75 m/sec
III	A-delta	5-30 m/sec
	B	3-15 m/sec
IV	C	.05-2 m/sec

The classification systems have been intermixed in the literature such that a C fiber may be used to refer to sensory or motor fiber with a conduction speed of approximately .05-2 meters per second.

It is important to understand that there is nothing mysterious about the names of these nerve fibers. Regardless of the label, the classification has been done according to axonal size.

Certain sizes of fibers do tend to be associated with particular types of receptors. In general, the following holds true:

A-alpha (I)	- proprioceptors
A-beta-gamma	- proprioceptors, exteroceptors
A-delta	- exteroceptors
C	- exteroceptors (mostly less complex "free nerve-ending" types)

55. The muscle spindle is one of several sensory receptors found in muscle and related connective tissue.   The muscle spindle is a highly complex receptor which is responsive to the length of the muscle and changes in that length.

    The muscle spindle consists of its own specialized muscle fibers encased within a connective tissue capsule.   There are two types of sensory nerve endings which innervate the muscle spindle: the primary and secondary afferent receptors.

    As movement occurs or a position is maintained the length of the muscle is monitored by the _____ _____.

muscle spindle

---

56. The muscle spindle is one type of sensory receptor in skeletal muscle.   It monitors muscle movements and through reflex pathways it assists in regulating them. This receptor would be classified as a proprioceptor.

    The muscle spindle is made up of two specialized types of muscle fibers; the **nuclear bag** fibers and the **nuclear chain** fibers.   Both of these fibers are called **intrafusal** muscle fibers.

    The first intrafusal muscle fiber has its nuclei grouped in the center as if they are in a bag, and is, therefore, called the _____ _____ fiber.

nuclear bag

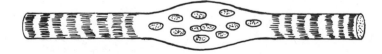

113

57. The second intrafusal muscle fiber has its nuclei arranged in series and has no swelling. It is, therefore, called the _____ _____ fiber.

nuclear chain

---

58. The fibers contained in the muscle spindle are called intrafusal muscle fibers. The fiber has contractile muscle elements at both ends. These elements are contiguous with the non-contractile portion (equatorial region) of the fibers in which the nuclei are contained.

Both the nuclear _____ and nuclear _____ are intra _____ muscle fibers.

bag
chain
fusal

EQUATORIAL REGION

---

59. Both the nuclear chain and nuclear bag fibers have _____ muscle elements at each end.

contractile

The center of the non-contractile area of the fiber is called the _____ region.

equatorial

60. The two intrafusal muscle fibers, nuclear _____ and nuclear _____, are encased in a connective tissue capsule.

bag
chain

_____

61. Each connective tissue capsule contains a varying ratio of nuclear bag to nuclear chain intrafusal muscle fibers depending on the animal and muscle investigated. In man there are approximately twice as many chain fibers as bag fibers; a generally accepted figure is two nuclear bag fibers and four nuclear chain fibers (Mountcastle, 1980).

In man, the connective tissue _____ contains more of the nuclear _____ fibers than it does nuclear _____ fibers.

capsule
chain
bag

_____

62. The connective tissue capsule is a membrane which is thickest in the center portion (or equatorial region) of the muscle spindle. The capsule becomes a thin membranous covering toward the polar regions of the intrafusal muscle fibers. Label the diagram.

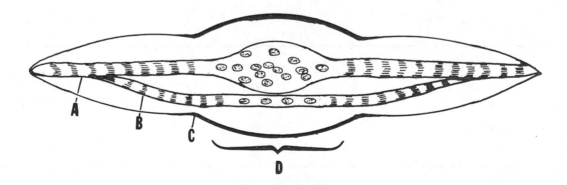

A.   nuclear chain
B.   nuclear bag
C.   connective tissue capsule
D.   equatorial region

63. Some authorities maintain that the nuclear chain intrafusal muscle fibers may be attached to the nuclear bag fibers and may also attach to the connective tissue _____ (Granit, 1970).

capsule

---

64. This sensory unit, called the **muscle spindle** is made up of two nuclear _____ fibers and four nuclear _____ fibers encased in a _____ _____ capsule.

This is one type of a _____ unit for skeletal muscle.

bag
chain
connective tissue
sensory

NOTE: Studies investigating **human** muscle spindles have shown that there are 2 to 14 intrafusal muscle fibers in one spindle. Other complexites were noted; muscle spindles are often arranged in tandem with a single nuclear bag fiber extending through the length of two such spindles (Swash and Fox, 1972).

It is useful to recognize that the human muscle spindle may be more complicated than is described in this volume, however, the details presented should be sufficient for a functional understanding of the subject.

---

65. The fibers contained in the muscle spindle are called _____ muscle fibers.

intrafusal

---

66. The nuclear chain fiber may be attached to the _____ _____ fiber.

nuclear bag

67. The muscle spindle is a _____ unit for skeletal muscle.

sensory

---

68. One end of the nuclear bag intrafusal muscle fiber is attached to the endomysium of an extrafusal muscle fiber. All connective tissue ultimately blends together and extends to the tendon.

In a skeletal muscle, the nuclear bag fiber of a muscle spindle is attached to the endomysium of one of its _____ muscle fibers.

extrafusal

ENDOMYSIUM   NUCLEAR CHAIN   NUCLEAR BAG

---

69. Muscle cells or fibers making up a muscle are referred to as _____ muscle fibers.

extrafusal

---

70. The bulk of each muscle is made up of these extrafusal fibers. They are arranged in parallel with those of the muscle spindle, the _____ muscle fibers.

intrafusal

117

71. Application of a force to two parallel structures will result in equal stress to the parallel parts.

If the extrafusal muscle fiber is stretched, the muscle spindle is stretched. If the extrafusal muscle fiber is unloaded (neither stretched nor contracting) the muscle spindle is unloaded.

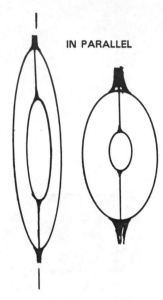

IN PARALLEL

STRETCH ONE AND THE
OTHER IS ALSO STRETCHED

This occurs because the extrafusal muscle fibers and the muscle spindle are arranged in _____.

parallel

_____

72. The muscle spindle is sensitive both to changes in length and to the velocity of such changes in the extra-_____ muscle fiber.

fusal

_____

73. One end of the nuclear bag intrafusal muscle fiber is attached to the endomysium of an extrafusal muscle fiber. All connective tissue ultimately blends together and extends to the _____.

tendon

74. One end of the nuclear bag intrafusal muscle fiber is also attached to the perimysium of the extrafusal muscle fiber. All layers of connective tissue of the muscle ultimately blend with the muscle tendon (Granit, 1970).

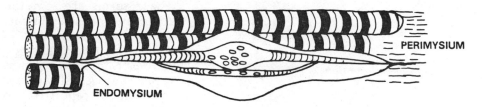

PERIMYSIUM

ENDOMYSIUM

Attached to the perimysium which surrounds a group of muscle cells are both the _____ and _____ muscle fibers.

extrafusal
intrafusal

75. Because both intrafusal and extrafusal fibers are attached to the perimysium and to each other, stretch applied to one must influence the other.

The muscle spindle and extrafusal muscle fibers are arranged in _____.

parallel

76. One end of the muscle spindle (nuclear bag fibers) is attached to the endomysium of the _____ _____ fiber.

extrafusal muscle

77. The other end of the nuclear bag fiber is usually attached to the _____.

perimysium

119

78. Each intrafusal muscle fiber has both sensory and motor innervation. First the sensory receptors will be considered.

Sensory nerve fibers have static and dynamic components.

These terms are sometimes confused with the terms tonic and phasic. In fact, many references use the terms interchangeably (Kandel, 1981; Bishop, 1982). The terms phasic and tonic are perhaps best utilized to describe such events as moving versus holding; rapid versus slow; and short or quick versus maintained, repetitive or continued. Standing for a long time is a tonic condition. Jumping is a phasic condition. If a motor neuron is tonically active, it maintains an output for an extended period.

A knee jerk is a _____ response.

phasic

_____

79. Stimuli or responses that are maintained or repetitive are considered tonic in nature.

Standing at attention for a long period of time is a _____ activity.

tonic

_____

80. Static and dynamic are terms we will use in this book to relate more specifically to the type of response of the sensory receptors in muscle and the motor fibers to the muscle spindle, which enhance the static and dynamic responses.

The unchanging length of a muscle is considered to be a _____ condition.

static

81. The rate of change of length or velocity is a measure of a _____ condition.

dynamic

___

82. A sustained repetitive motor output from the alpha motor neuron is a _____ response.

tonic

___

83. The muscle spindle is sensitive both to the length of the extrafusal muscle and to the rate, or velocity, of change in length. Some sensory receptors will be more sensitive to changes in velocity while others will be more sensitive to muscle _____.

length

___

84. Sensory receptors which respond to the length of a muscle could be called _____ receptors.

static

___

85. Some of the terminology used to describe the muscle spindle has changed in recent years. The following chart may help orient those who are familiar with previously used terms.

Classification	Newer Term	Previous Term
Ia	primary afferent	annulospiral
II	secondary afferent	flower spray

As opposed to the older term flower spray, the receptors classified as II are now referred to as _____ afferents.

secondary

86. Label the following diagram:

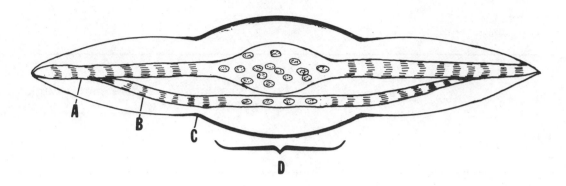

a. nuclear bag fiber
b. nuclear chain fiber
c. connective tissue capsule
d. equatorial region

---

87. The extrafusal muscle fibers and the muscle spindle are arranged in _____.

parallel

---

88. Each intrafusal muscle has both _____ and _____ innervation.

sensory
motor

---

89. Stimuli or responses that are maintained or repetitive are considered to be _____ in nature.

tonic

122

90. The primary afferent nerve fiber (Ia) is one sensory component of the muscle spindle. In older books it is referred to as the annulospiral fiber because it is wrapped in spiral fashion around the center portion of the muscle spindle.

    The arrow points to the Ia, annulospiral, or _____ _____ nerve fiber.

primary afferent

91. The Ia classification comes from the axon or fiber size associated with the annulospiral receptor. The axon is the largest in its classification. Thus the axon is an A-_____ fiber.

alpha

92. The Ia receptor is also referred to as the _____ or _____ _____ receptor.

annulospinal
primary afferent

93. To avoid confusion with classification systems that utilize Roman numerals, we will refer to this receptor as the primary afferent receptor. The symbol Ia will appear in parentheses because you may encounter this label in the literature.

The primary sensory receptors of both the nuclear chain and nuclear bag fibers are served by branches from one primary nerve fiber.

These are separate receptors but are components of a single nerve fiber. These primary afferent fibers are also called _____ or _____ fibers.

Ia
annulospiral

---

94. Each spindle has a single primary afferent (Ia) nerve fiber that subdivides and sends spirals around the equatorial region of all intrafusal muscle fibers. This includes both nuclear _____ and _____ muscle fibers.

bag
chain

---

95. Histochemical and ultrastructural studies have shown that there are actually two types of nuclear bag fibers. One has properties which are functionally dynamic and the other possesses static properties (Boyd, 1976; Saito, et.al., 1977).

These fibers have been called the _____ nuclear bag and _____ nuclear bag fibers.

static
dynamic

---

96. Nuclear bag fibers may be classified as either _____ or _____.

static
dynamic

124

97. The primary afferent nerve fiber from the dynamic nuclear bag intrafusal muscle fiber is the most responsive to the rate of change in muscle length.

We could, therefore, label it as a _____ receptor.

dynamic

98. As the extrafusal muscle changes to a new length, the receptor which monitors this change would be considered a _____ receptor.

dynamic

99. When the change to a new length is maintained, the receptor which monitors this length would be considered a _____ receptor.

static

100. As you might expect, the static primary receptor is associated with the _____ nuclear bag fiber.

static

101. Is the dynamic Ia component of the primary afferent (Ia) nerve fibers labeled 1 or 2?

I

102. This dynamic receptor is primarily sensitive to the velocity (or rate) of change in length. It will respond to a **quick stretch** of the extrafusal muscle and by reflex action will produce a **quick contraction** of the extrafusal muscle. This is why it is referred to as a _____ receptor.

dynamic

103. If the muscle spindle in the biceps muscle is subjected to a quick stretch anywhere in the range of motion, it will respond by producing a _____ _____ of the biceps.

quick or phasic contraction

104. A quick stretch should activate the dynamic component of the _____ _____.

primary afferent receptor

105. In the biceps muscle, if the primary afferent receptor (Ia) is quickly stretched (such as by a tendon tap) it sends impulses to the spinal cord which travel to the synaptic junction between the sensory axon and motor neuron to the biceps.

The stimulation of the alpha motor neurons causes motor units in the biceps to contract (shorten), which relieves the load on the muscle spindle and decreases the number of impulses transmitted by the primary (Ia) fiber.

The alpha motor neuron is the motor supply to the _____ muscle fiber.

extrafusal

---

106. Label the components of the reflex arc.

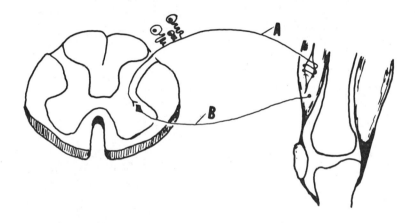

A - primary afferent fiber
B - Alpha motor neuron

---

107. The primary reflex arc may be considered a functional cycle.

If the primary receptor is activated by stretch, the number of impulses its axon transmits increases. This activation facilitates the alpha motor neuron in the spinal cord.

If the threshold is reached, the alpha motor neuron fires. Alpha motor neuron activation causes the extrafusal muscle fibers to _____.

contract

108. The primary (Ia) receptors respond to a quick stretch to the muscle and produce a _____ contraction.

quick or phasic

---

109. In the following diagram, a (+) means stretch applied or neuron excited, and (-) indicates lack of stimulation or inhibition. Depicted below is a cycle that occurs when stretch is applied to a primary receptor.

*Indicates starting point.

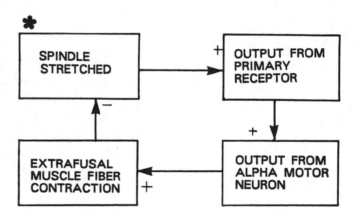

Stretch will excite the primary receptor which, in turn, may result in excitation of the alpha _____ neuron.

motor

---

110. The motor neuron fires when _____ is reached.

threshold

111. Indicate excitation (+) and inhibition (-) and fill in the boxes where appropriate.

*Indicates starting point.

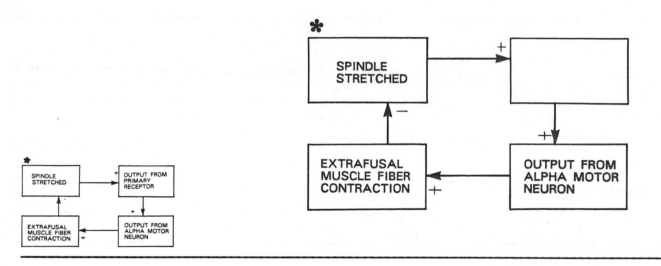

---

112. When Sherrington originally did his classical work examining reflexes in decerebrate cats he found that when he attempted to forcefully flex the rigidly extended limb, the limb resisted the force by active contraction of the extensor muscles.

He, therefore, called the response the **myotatic** (Greek for extended muscle) or the **stretch** reflex.

There are two components to the stretch reflex. The first is the phasic component. This is usually short and relatively intense (Kandel, 1981).

A "tendon jerk" may be classified as a _____ _____ reflex.

phasic stretch

---

113. The second component of the stretch reflex is the _____ component.

tonic

129

114. The tonic stretch reflex is less intense than the phasic stretch reflex and lasts _____.

longer

---

115. In the tonic stretch reflex the contraction lasts as long as the stretch. The tonic stretch reflex is thought to be most important in the maintainence of posture.

It lasts longer than the phasic stretch reflex and is less _____.

intense

---

116. Phasic stretch reflexes are triggered by movement. Movement of a joint causes a change in muscle _____ (Kandel, 1981).

length

---

117. The tonic component of stretch reflexes is elicited by a steady _____ to the muscles.

stretch

---

118. The nerve fiber which is responsible for monosynaptic myotatic spinal level reflexes such as the knee jerk is the _____.

primary (Ia)

119. Fill in the boxes to complete the functional cycle. Designate excitation (+) and inhibition (-).

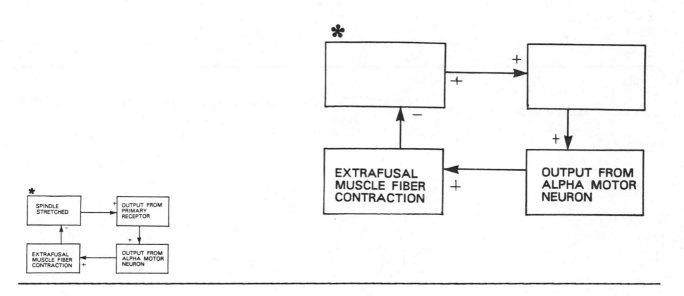

120. The primary receptors from the nuclear chain and static nuclear bag intrafusal muscle fibers provide the static component of the afferent nerve fiber. This component responds to a **maintained stretch** and reflexly produces a **maintained contraction.**

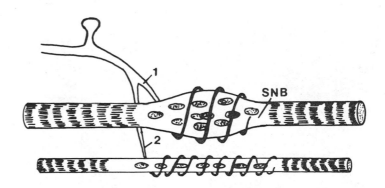

The fibers which are innervated by the static primary receptor are labeled _____.

1 and 2

131

121. The response to **maintained** stimuli and the production of **maintained** contractions involve the primary afferent (Ia) receptor. These maintained contractions contribute to a _____ stretch reflex.

tonic

---

122. The primary fibers make monosynaptic connections with the alpha motor neurons to their own muscle. Label the parts of the monosynaptic reflex arc.

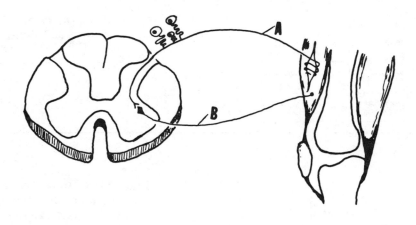

A. Primary afferent (Ia)
B. Alpha motor neuron

---

123. In review, fill in the boxes and indicate excitation and inhibition.

*Indicates starting point.

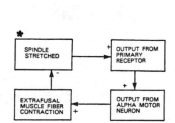

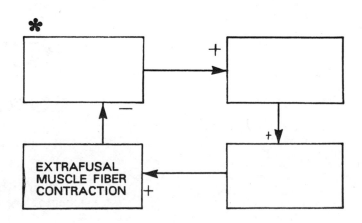

124. If the extrafusal muscle contracts it relieves the load on the _____ _____.

muscle spindle

---

125. It is imperative that you understand that the input from **one** primary afferent (Ia) fiber is not sufficient to activate the alpha motor neuron. One synapse provides only approximately two percent of the input needed to activate the motor neuron (Bishop, 1982).

We have been referring to the input from single primary (Ia) fibers; however, motor cell depolarization requires _____ inputs.

multiple
or
more than 1

---

126. When the primary afferent (Ia) fiber enters the spinal cord, it branches. Some of the branches ascend to higher centers which we will consider later.

We used to believe that at the spinal cord level the primary fiber produced limited branching to impinge perhaps on a few select motor neurons to a homonymous muscle.

Animal studies on the cat now show that apparently a single primary (Ia) afferent may send terminals to **all** of the cells in that motor neuron pool Thus, the distribution of primary afferents to the muscle from which it originates (homonymous) is quite extensive. A single primary afferent fiber will be distributed to 71-100 percent of the motor neurons in the motor neuron pool (Mendell and Henneman, 1971; Nelson and Mendell, 1979).

If there are 300 motor neurons in the pool to the gastrocnemius muscle, a single primary sensory fiber may have as many as _____ terminals.

300

127. If other inputs are not active, however, a single primary afferent (Ia) terminal is not sufficient to _____ the anterior horn cell.

activate

---

128. A single primary afferent (Ia) fiber also sends terminals to many of the motor neurons of the synergists of its own muscle. The percentage of terminals to each of the synergistic motor neuron pools range from 42 to 74 percent.

A single primary afferent (Ia) fiber has many _____.

terminals

---

129. A single primary afferent fiber projects to most, if not all, of its homonomous muscle motor neurons and to a large percentage of the neurons which innervate its _____.

synergists

---

130. The excititory potentials (EPSPs) generated in the motor neuron to the homonymous muscle are larger than those generated by the same primary fiber to the cell bodies of the synergists. This finding indicates that stretch reflexes are best developed in the muscle which has been _____.

stretched

---

131. The nuclear chain fiber is innervated by a _____ receptor.

static

132. Recall that there are at least three types of motor units. The primary afferent receptors produce the strongest effects on the type I motor units.

You might expect that the primary receptors have their weakest influence on the type _____ motor units.

IIB

---

133. We will continue to refer to muscle spindle receptors in the singular sense relative to causing muscle contraction. You will, however, remember that the present level of facilitation of the cell will determine how much additional input is necessary to activate it. More than likely, a motor neuron will not be activated by a _____ _____ fiber.

single primary (Ia)

---

134. The muscle spindle response is said to be excititory to that muscle, if it produces excitatory potentials in the homonymous motor neurons. This excitation may or may not be sufficient to cause a muscle to _____.

contract

---

135. The dynamic component of the primary (Ia) nerve fiber is thus _____ to its own muscle.

excitatory

136. The static component of the primary afferent (Ia) nerve fiber is also excitatory to _____ _____ muscle.

its own

---

137. This phenomenon is referred to as autogenic facilitation. This simply means that an afferent nerve from a particular muscle excites or produces a contraction in that same _____.

muscle

---

138. The primary afferent (Ia) nerve fibers also have a connection to the antagonist and this connection is inhibitory. This phenomenon is referred to as reciprocal inhibition.

If the primary afferent (Ia) receptor within the biceps muscle is stretched, it causes the biceps to be _____ and the triceps to be _____.

excited
inhibited

---

139. The primary afferent receptor, therefore, produces autogenic _____.

excitation

---

140. Through reciprocal innervation the primary afferent receptor is _____ to its antagonists.

inhibitory

141. The static component of the primary receptor is excitatory to its own muscle and inhibitory to its antagonist. This also occurs with the primary (Ia) _____ component.

dynamic

142. The static component of the primary afferent (Ia) receptor in the biceps muscle, for instance, responds to a maintained stretch and facilitates a contraction of the biceps which is _____.

maintained

The triceps is thus _____.

inhibited

This inhibition is due to the phenomenon of _____ innervation.

reciprocal

143. The primary afferent fiber is responsive to the length of the muscle and the changes in length.

It is also documented that the primary afferent endings are very sensitive to vibration, particularly when applied to the tendon (Granit, 1970).

Primary afferent fibers of the muscle spindle can be selectively activated with _____.

vibration

144. If the vibration is maintained it will stimulate the _____ afferent component.

static

145. The primary afferent (Ia) receptor produces _____ excitation.

autogenetic

---

146. The primary afferent (Ia) fiber produces antagonist _____.

inhibition

---

147. One or more interneurons (small or short neuron situated between incoming and outgoing fibers in the spinal cord) must be present in any reflex circuit involving inhibition from Ia fibers or any other fibers.

Because of the extra synapse, inhibition requires more time than excitation.

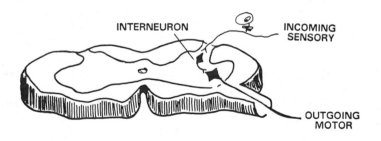

Each interneuron provides an extra synapse in the chain of neurons, therefore, inhibitory responses take more time to occur than do _____ responses.

monosynaptic
or
excitatory

148. Label the parts of the primary receptor mediated reflex.

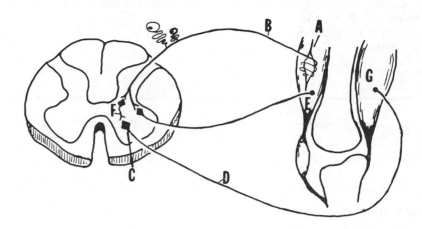

A. Primary receptor
B. Primary fiber (sensory)
C. Motor neuron (AHC alpha)
D. Axon (motor)
E. Homonymous muscle
F. Interneuron
G. Antagonist muscle

---

149. In review, fill in the boxes and indicate facilitation or inhibition.

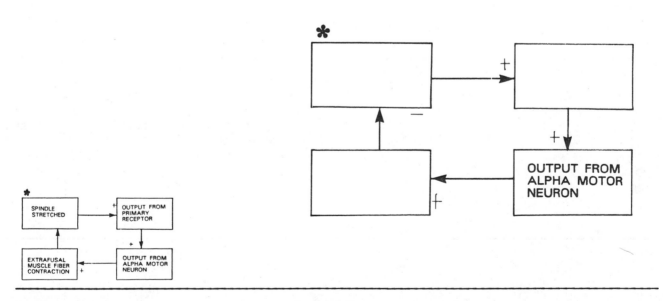

OUTPUT FROM ALPHA MOTOR NEURON

✱

SPINDLE STRETCHED → + → OUTPUT FROM PRIMARY RECEPTOR

EXTRAFUSAL MUSCLE FIBER CONTRACTION ← + ← OUTPUT FROM ALPHA MOTOR NEURON

---

150. Primary receptors (Ia) produce excitation in the _____ muscle.

same or homonymous

139

151. Primary afferent receptors (Ia) are responsive to
_____
_____ .

muscle length and
changes in muscle
length

152. The primary receptors (Ia) are also selectively
responsive to _____ .

vibration

153. Muscle spindle receptors are responsible for
_____ reflexes.

stretch

154. Stretch reflexes may have both _____ and
_____ components.

phasic
tonic

155. The phasic stretch reflex or portion of the reflex may
be best triggered by abrupt _____ .

movement

steady stretch

156. The tonic stretch reflex or portion of the reflex is sustained by a _____ _____ to the muscles.

phasic stretch

157. A knee jerk reflex is a _____ _____ reflex.

tonic stretch

158. Postural control is most strongly supported by _____ _____ reflexes.

synergists

159. The primary afferent (Ia) fiber sends terminals to its own muscle and to its _____ as well.

synergists

160. The stretch reflexes are best developed in the muscle that was stretched as opposed to its _____.

SUMMARY

The muscle spindle is a sensory receptor located in parallel with the extrafusal muscle fibers. The spindle consists of two types of intrafusal muscle fibers: the nuclear chain and nuclear bag fibers. There are two types of nuclear bag fibers, the static and dynamic nuclear bag fibers. The intrafusal fibers are encased within a connective tissue capsule.

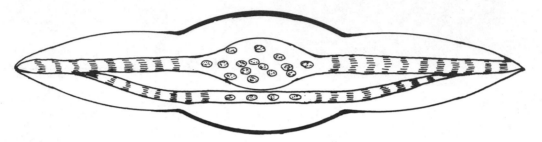

The muscle spindle is innervated by two types of receptors. The receptor thus far described is the primary afferent fiber (Ia). It consists of a spiral ending which is wrapped around the equatorial region of the nuclear bag and the nuclear chain fibers.

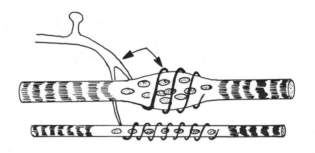

When the extrafusal muscle fibers are stretched the intrafusal fibers are also stretched, which provides an excitatory stimulus to the primary afferent receptors. Thus, the muscle spindle is sensitive to the change in muscle length and the rate of that change.

The primary afferent fiber from the dynamic nuclear bag intrafusal muscle fiber (dynamic component) is the most responsive to the rate of change in muscle length. The dynamic primary receptor mediates the phasic stretch reflex which is elicited best by the application of abrupt movement.

The primary receptor from the nuclear chain and the static nuclear bag fibers is the static component of the receptor and it responds to a maintained stretch. This portion of the receptor mediates the tonic stretch reflex in which a maintained contraction persists as long as the stretch is present.

142

The primary (Ia) receptor is excitatory to its own muscle and inhibitory to its antagonist. The latter phenomenon is called reciprocal inhibition.

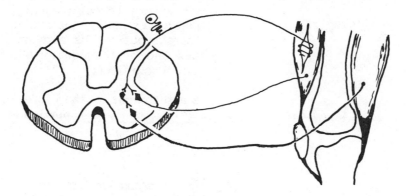

Experimental evidence indicates that one primary receptor sends terminals to all of the motor neurons in the motor neuron pool. It also sends terminals to 42 to 74 percent of the motor neurons to the synergists.

The input from one primary ending to a motor neuron is usually not sufficient to activate that neuron. The present level of facilitation of the neuron cell body along with simultaneous input from all sources determines whether the neuron will be activated.

The primary endings are highly sensitive to vibration.

161. The secondary (II) or "flower spray" ending is the other sensory receptor found in the muscle spindle. It innervates mainly the nuclear chain fiber. Part of it "sprays out" at its attachment and is located at either end of the equatorial region of the nuclear chain muscle fiber.

The attachment is, therefore, relatively close to the _____ portion of the muscle fibers.

contractile

162. Many texts refer to the secondary receptor with the symbol II. This receptor has a II or "A-gamma" size axon which is likely why it was assigned this symbol in the first place. To avoid confusion we will refer to this receptor as the "secondary" receptor rather than "_____" receptor.

II

163. The secondary receptor has an _____ size axon.

A-gamma

144

164. The secondary (II) receptors were at one time called "flower spray" because a portion of the ending sprays out near the junction of the contractile element with the equatorial region. This receptor primarily serves the nuclear _____ fiber.

chain

---

165. The secondary (II) receptors are located primarily on nuclear _____ fibers.

chain

---

166. The secondary receptor (II) responds to a maintained stretch and reflexly produces a maintained contraction.

The secondary receptor (II) is not sensitive to vibration and is relatively insensitive to the velocity of muscle contraction.

The secondary receptor is sensitive to changes in muscle _____ and produces _____ responses.

length
maintained or tonic

---

167. Secondary (II) receptors are sensitive to changes in _____ _____.

muscle length

145

velocity
vibration

168. Secondary receptors are not sensitive to _____ or _____.

---

169. At one time physiologists believed that secondary (II) receptors were excitatory **only** to flexor muscles. Thus if the secondary receptor was located in an extensor muscle and was activated the extensor would be _____.

inhibited

---

170. According to this view autogenic excitation would only occur if the secondary receptor was activated in a _____ muscle.

flexor

---

171. If receptors within extensor muscles are to be inhibitory to their own muscles an interneuron must be present within the reflex circuit. Sensory neurons are all excitatory, therefore, all monosynaptic reflexes must also be _____.

excitatory

---

172. At one time physiologic evidence suggested that secondary receptors made only multisynaptic reflex connections. If this arrangement were true, it would be possible for reflexes mediated by the secondary receptors to produce autogenic inhibition of the extensor muscles.

The primary receptor (Ia) produces autogenic _____.

excitation

173. Current evidence clearly shows that the secondary receptor (II) also makes monosynaptic reflex connections (Matthews, 1969; Mountcastle, 1980). Under these conditions the secondary receptor cannot produce autogenic inhibition and will produce autogenic _____.

excitation

---

174. If secondary receptors within extensor muscles make monosynaptic connections with the alpha motor neurons the extensors will be _____ and the flexors _____.

excited
inhibited

---

175. The older view of the physiology of secondary receptors was that they were **always** specifically excitatory to _____ muscles and inhibitory to _____ muscles.

flexor
extensor

---

176. There is new evidence that the secondary receptors make at least some monosynaptic connections as does the _____ receptor.

primary (Ia)

---

177. Therefore, the secondary receptor may also produce _____ of its own muscle.

excitation

178. Other evidence also indicates that the secondary response supports the stretch reflex along with the _____ receptor.

primary (Ia)

179. Because of its sensitivity to static stimuli, the secondary receptor will contribute to the _____ stretch reflex.

tonic

180. Monosynaptic connections of the secondary (II) receptor produces autogenic _____.

excitation

181. These secondary afferent fibers will produce inhibition in the _____.

antagonist

182. The threshold to stretch of the secondary receptor is only slightly higher than that of the _____ receptor.

primary (Ia)

183. Although the secondary receptor has only a slightly higher threshold to stretch than the primary (Ia) receptor, when the muscle is in a shortened state its discharge rate is very slow.

The secondary receptor is responsive throughout the range. However, when the muscle is stretched near its physiological limits, the secondary (II) receptor discharge rate is greater than that from the primary (Ia) ending.

If the secondary receptor (II) is to fire at its greatest rate, the muscle must be placed on a maximum _____ (Barker, 1962).

stretch

---

184. Multisynaptic connections of the secondary receptor may be specifically excitatory to _____.

flexors

---

185. The best type of stretch for activating the secondary receptor is _____ stretch.

steady or
maintained

---

186. Studies on the projection of secondary receptors are much less clear than those of the primary receptors (Ia). It does appear from the literature that they do terminate on more than one anterior horn cell but do not seem to have as wide a distribution as do the _____ receptors.

primary (Ia)

187. There are one to five secondary receptors per spindle. Activity arising in them most likely exerts effects on the motor neurons through several reflex pathways such as the stretch reflex and possibly the flexor reflexes.

The secondary receptor does contribute to the _____ reflex.

stretch

---

188. It is apparent that both the primary and secondary receptors make multisynaptic connections with the motor neurons as well as monosynaptic reflex connections (Houk & Rymer, 1981; Stuart, 1981).

It is likely that some of the secondary receptors in any muscle may be specifically excitatory to _____.

flexors

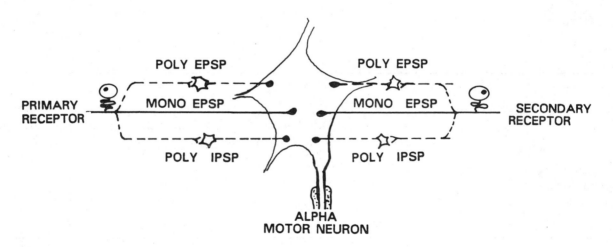

---

189. The primary receptor (Ia) probably also makes multisynaptic connections as well as _____ ones.

monosynaptic

190. It is likely that some primary sensory multisynaptic circuits may be _____ to their own muscle.

inhibitory

---

191. It is apparent that secondary receptors make both _____ and _____ connections

monosynaptic
multisynaptic

---

192. It is clear that the secondary receptor contributes to the tonic stretch reflex through its _____ connections.

monosynaptic

---

193. It is possible that some contributions from the secondary receptors **may** be specifically excitatory to _____ and inhibitory to _____.

flexors
extensors

---

194. The older view of the secondary receptor as being exclusively excitatory to flexors has been disproven.

That some of these receptors may still perform this function has not been _____.

disproven

195. The secondary (II) receptor fiber is also one potential contributor to the "clasp knife" reflex which was long thought to be the domain of the Golgi tendon organ which we will discuss later (Kandel, 1981).

The clasp knife reflex is found in patients with spasticity. In spasticity there is a marked resistance to passive stretch. If this stretch is continued, however, there may be a sudden loss of resistance to the stretch.

This loss of resistance is a length-dependent inhibition. The secondary (II) receptors are the most effective muscle _____ monitors.

length

---

196. With the clasp-knife reflex, the greater the static length of the muscle the greater the inhibition produced which will decrease the resistance to further _____.

stretch

---

197. The secondary receptor (II) is sensitive to muscle length and contributes to the following reflexes: (1)_____, (2)_____, and (3)_____.

tonic stretch
clasp-knife
flexor

---

198. Some investigations support the classical concept of the secondary receptor function. Studies in humans who have spinal cord injuries are in agreement with the findings in the spinal cat (Burke, et.al., 1970; 1971).

That is, in spinal man, secondary receptors may be excitatory specifically to _____.

flexors

199. Studies of patients with injuries higher in the central nervous system do not show the same responses (Andrews, et.al., 1972; 1973a; 1973b; Ashby & Burke, 1971).

The findings in these patients are variable and have not been fully explained. The predominant reflexes in which the secondary receptor participates are mediated by spinal cord interneurons (Urbscheit, 1979).

If the higher levels of the nervous system are damaged there will be marked alteration in the activity of the interneurons.

Certain lesions may activate one reflex response of the secondary receptor circuit and other lesions may inhibit the circuits (Urbscheit, 1979).

It is apparent that the secondary receptors can participate in a variety of reflex actions depending upon the integrity and state of the _____.

CNS

---

200. One should not expect that the reflex response will be the same in all _____.

patients

---

201. It is unlikely that the same treatment approach will _____ all patients.

benefit
or
help

---

202. For the moment, we have completed our discussion of the **afferent** components of the muscle spindle. There are also **motor** components to the muscle spindle.

The primary (Ia) and secondary (II) endings are _____ components.

sensory or
afferent

153

SUMMARY

The secondary or flower spray ending (II) is found primarily on the nuclear chain fiber. It is located at the equatorial region close to the contractile portion of these intrafusal muscle fibers.

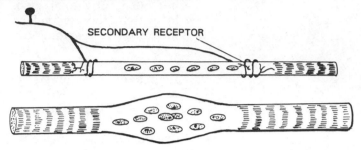

The secondary receptor is is relatively insensitive to vibration and to the velocity of muscle contraction. This receptor is most responsive to change in muscle length. Because secondary output continues with maintained stretch, it can be concluded that the secondary ending contributes to the tonic stretch reflex along with the primary ending.

The secondary ending will fire at its greatest rate when the length of the muscle is near its physiological limits.

Physiological evidence gathered from studies of the flexor reflex afferents was at one time interpreted in such a way as to lead us to believe that the secondary ending was always specifically excitatory to flexors and inhibitory to extensors no matter where it was located. Much clinical intervention has been based on this assumption.

We now know that the secondary ending does have monosynaptic connections with the motor neurons and is, therefore, capable of autogenic excitation regardless of whether it is located in a flexor or extensor muscle.

There are A beta-gamma (II) size fibers in muscle nerves which, when activated, result in the net inhibition of extensors and facilitation of flexors. It is not known whether some of these fibers actually come from the muscle spindle. If they do it can be said that there are also polysynaptic connections from the secondary ending which may contribute to the flexor reflex as well as to the tonic stretch reflex.

Evidence in human studies suggests that secondary receptors particiate in a variety of reflex responses. In pathological conditions different responses may occur depending upon the type and location of the lesion within the central nervous system.

203. Another sensory organ associated with muscle is the Golgi tendon organ (GTO). It is located in the musculo-tendinous junction both at the muscle origin and the insertion, and is sensitive to tension (Granit, 1970).

Label components of muscle spindle illustrated.

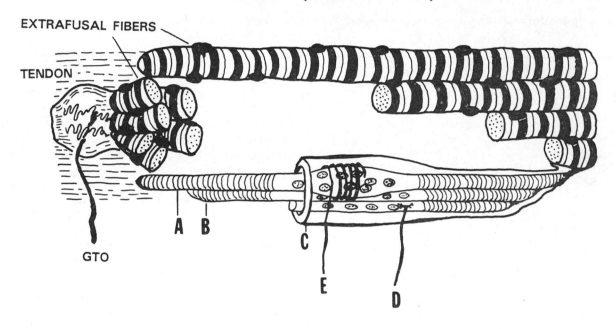

EXTRAFUSAL FIBERS

TENDON

GTO

A B

C

E

D

A   nuclear bag fiber
B   nuclear chain fiber
C   connective tissue capsule
D   secondary receptor
E   primary receptor
     (dynamic component)

204. The muscle spindle reponds to changes in muscle length and to the rate or velocity of such changes. The GTO is a receptor that is sensitive to muscle _____.

tension

205. The GTO capsule is attached to about 10 extrafusal muscle fibers. These fibers belong to different motor units. Thus if the motor unit firing has a fiber represented in the GTO capsule, the tension produced by that motor unit will be monitored. The GTO is thus arranged in series with extrafusal muscle fibers (Granit, 1970).

    The muscle spindle is arranged in _____ with extrafusal muscle fibers.

parallel

---

206. The Golgi tendon organ is a slender capsule through which a discrete number of skeletal muscle fibers enter as if through a funnel-like collar. The connective tissue surrounding the muscle fibers coalesces into bundles which become braided with one another.

    The afferent fiber enters the capsule in the middle of the capsule and gives rise to many branches. The axonal branches become twisted within the collagen bundle braids. When the extrafusal muscle fibers contract the collagen bundles are straightened. This straightening compresses the axon terminals, causing them to fire (Kandel, 1981).

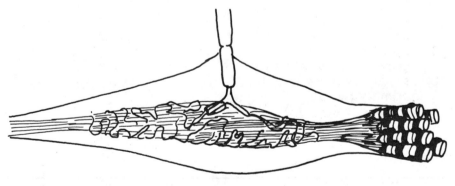

GOLGI TENDON ORGAN

Very few motor units are represented in any one _____ _____ _____.

Golgi tendon organ

156

207. Because the GTO is arranged in series, it may be stimulated by **passive** stretch on the tendon through its muscle, or by **contraction** of the muscle. The GTO has a very high threshold to passive stretch, but may be so sensitive to muscle **contraction** as to pick up tension activity from a **single motor unit.**

The GTO is more sensitive to _____ _____ than to stretch.

muscle contraction

_____

208. The relative insensitivity of the GTO to passive stretch most likely relates to the large amount of stretch which would be required to place much tension on the tendon when passively elongating the muscle. Thus the GTO would appear to have a high threshold to passive stretch.

Because the GTO has muscle fibers representing certain motor units, the GTO would likely monitor the contraction of that unit and thus appear to be more sensitive to muscle contraction than to passive _____.

stretch

_____

209. The GTO (fiber type Ib) is very sensitive to tension produced by _____ _____.

muscle contraction

_____

210. The GTO is arranged in _____ with the extrafusal muscle fibers.

series

211. The Golgi tendon organ causes what is called auto-genic inhibition. The primary and most secondary receptors produce autogenic _____.

excitation

---

212. The GTO is inhibitory to its own muscle and also excitatory to its antagonist. If the GTO in the biceps muscle is stimulated, it will _____ the biceps and _____ the triceps.

inhibit
excite

---

213. Note that GTO receptors have axons in the I or A-alpha category. The size of these axons are slightly smaller than those of the primary afferent (Ia) and are referred to as Ib. Again, we will place this label in parenthesis as you will encounter it in the literature.

In some references, the GTO may be identified as _____.

Ib

---

214. The GTO does not appear to make any monosynaptic connections. All connections to motor neurons are made through interneurons.

In terms of time, compared to primary afferent (Ia) reflexes, GTO mediated reflexes will be _____.

slower

215. Label the interneurons in the diagram as to whether they are excitatory (+) or inhibitory (-).

1 -
2 -
3 +

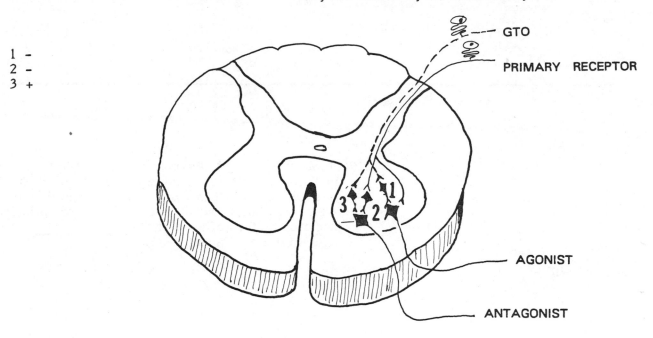

GTO

PRIMARY RECEPTOR

AGONIST

ANTAGONIST

---

216. The GTO has some other features that are strikingly different from the primary receptors in specific, and the muscle spindle in general.

The central connections of the Golgi tendon organ (Ib) are much more widespread than those of the _____ fiber.

primary

---

217. GTO (Ib) afferent effects are very strong in extensor muscles and, in fact, are relatively weak in flexor muscles.

Additionally, in comparison to the primary receptor (Ia) ending, the GTO (Ib) afferents produce much more _____ effects.

widespread

218. GTO afferent (Ib) effects are the strongest in the
_____ muscles.

extensor

---

219. Physiologists used to consider the GTO as the
mediator of the clasp-knife reflex.   While it is
possible that the GTO makes some contribution, most
likely the initiation of the reflex, the principal
mediator of the reflex is the _____
afferent ending (Kandel, 1981).

secondary (II)

---

220. The activity of the primary fiber (Ia) or receptor
would implicate it as the **main** receptor responsible
for the phenomenon of _____
inhibition.

reciprocal

---

221. Researchers believe that the GTO system could act
as a tension feedback system. Increases in tension
beyond a desirable level would produce negative
feedback from the GTO and this feedback would
inhibit any further development of _____.

tension

222. It is not fully understood just how a muscle functions normally if inhibition is increased as muscle contraction is increased. It has been postulated, and fairly well documented, that the GTO tension receptor is the damping (protective) mechanism against over contraction or stretch of the muscle (Granit, 1970).

The protective mechanism is probably the GTO, a _____ receptor.

tension

---

223. If the tension level is decreasing as in the case of muscle fatigue, an opposite function occurs. The tendon organ would be less activated because of the decreased tension so the motor neurons would receive less _____.

inhibition

---

224. If there were less autogenic inhibition on the motor neurons, more tension would develop which would compensate for the _____.

fatigue

---

225. Interneurons within the GTO (Ib) afferent reflex pathways also receive short-latency excitation from low threshold cutaneous and joint afferents.

In a situation in which the limb movement met an obstacle these afferents might excite the GTO reflex pathways which would inhibit the muscle and reduce further force against the _____ (Kandel, 1981).

obstacle

161

226. The above interaction could be considered to be a protective mechanism.

Cutaneous and joint afferents could assist in limiting the range of a movement by exciting the GTO _____ _____.

reflex pathways

227. Another possible function of the GTO may be to signal increased levels of tension as the joint reaches the mechanical limit of its range. In this case, at the end of a flexion or extension movement, the GTO (Ib) fiber inhibition would decrease the terminal force of the muscle and facilitate protective contraction in the antagonist.

This mechanism undoubtedly helps to protect the _____.

joint

228. Whether activation of the GTO will actually inhibit each motor unit depends on the muscle (flexor or extensor) in which it is located, and the "bias" or level of activity of the interneuron pool and the type and sensitivity of the motor neuron upon which it fires.

Inhibition by the GTO, then, depends on the type of muscle innervated by the GTO and the "bias" of the _____ _____ and _____ pools.

motor neuron
interneuron

229. The GTO appears to be more sensitive to muscle contraction than to muscle _____.

length
or
elongation

162

230. Changes in muscle length do not affect the GTO (Ib) significantly because the receptors are located in relatively inelastic connective tissue capsules. It has been found, however, that if active contraction occurs when the muscle is lengthened and the ends are relatively "fixed" or stable, very vigorous firing occurs (Mountcastle, 1980).

An example of such a condition is when the soleus muscle is lengthened during a weight bearing squat and the position is maintained.

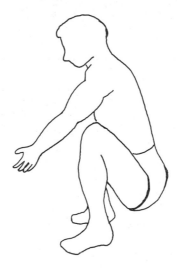

Thus, a stretch and contraction that are present simultaneously in a relatively fixed or static muscle length will result in a large output of the _____.

GTO

---

231. It has been postulated that the GTO is responsible for the stretch relief of some muscle cramps. In a painful cramp, when the muscle is fully shortened there is no tension produced on the tendon and the GTO is silent.

If the contracting muscle is stretched out to a long length, the tendon organs are activated and produce a relaxation which will relieve the cramp by strongly _____ the muscle (Mountcastle, 1980).

inhibiting

232. The GTO pathway involves the activation of interneurons. The algebraic sum of all excitatory impulses (+) and all inhibitory impulses (-) of an interneuron pool or circuit at a given moment determines whether the threshold will be reached and the cell being acted upon will fire. This is what is meant by "bias" of an interneuron pool (Granit, 1970).

The algebraic sum of all impulses on the interneuron pool determines whether the _____ will be reached.

threshold

---

233. If the (+s) are greater than (-s) at a given moment, the interneuron pool is "_____" toward facilitation.

biased

---

234. The interneuron pool regulates all impulses to the alpha motor neuron except those from the mono-synapic reflex arc. These pools have extremely complex circuits and controls, and act differently on flexors than extensors. Therefore, mechanisms such as the GTO are difficult to evaluate.

The regulation of most impulses to the neurons is by the _____ _____.

interneuron pool

---

235. The GTO mechanism has a multisynaptic pathway which indicates it may have a number of _____ in the reflex pathway.

interneurons

236. To classify the GTO as participating in either tonic or phasic reflexes is difficult. As it responds to muscle tension as well as to the rate of change in tension, it would be easiest to think of it as being both static and dynamic in nature.

The GTO responds to the amount of tension and rate of change in _____.

tension

---

237. It is perhaps wise, at this point, to think of the GTO as having both _____ and _____ functions.

static
dynamic

---

238. The GTO can be put in the functional cycle. Label any blank boxes.

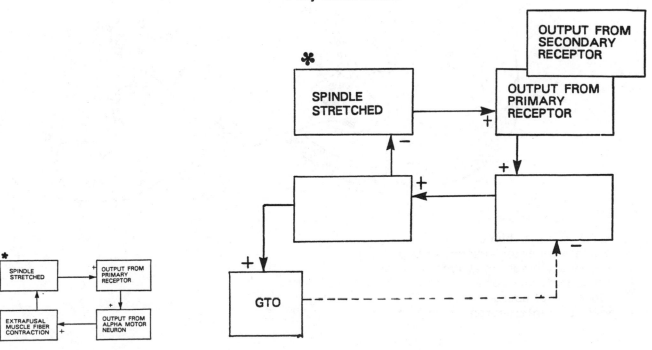

239. The GTO (Ib) will inhibit its own muscle and excite its antagonists.

This is due to the same phenomenon mentioned previously, i.e. _____ innervation.

reciprocal

---

240. The GTO (Ib) and some secondary (II) fiber pathways have multiple synapses, although in this text we will use one interneuron to represent inhibition. Multiple interneurons will not be depicted.

The GTO (I___) has a synapse in the spinal cord with the alpha motor neuron supplying its own muscle and that supplying its antagonist.

b

Label the sensory and motor components in the diagram and how each affects the agonist and antagonist. (Use + and -).

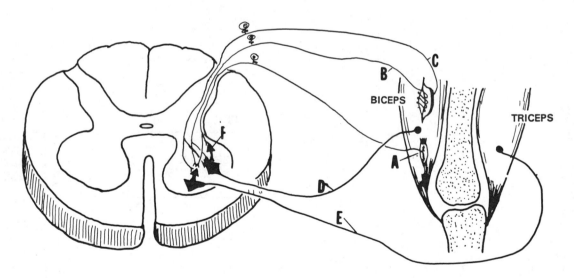

A GTO -triceps +biceps
B primary receptor +triceps -biceps
C secondary receptor +triceps -biceps
D alpha motor neuron
E alpha motor neuron
F inhibitory interneuron

INTERNEURONS

241. Most synaptic connections in the central nervous system involve interneurons. Although in the minority, the primary afferents and their monosynaptic connections are probably the best known because their accessibility has made them the most studied of all synapses.

Most of the synapses to the motor neuron, are with _____.

interneurons

---

242. Interneurons play an important role in controlling transmission of information. These cells form indirect divergent and convergent loops which are superimposed on more direct pathways.

Neural activity which reaches a particular neuron by a direct pathway will also evoke activity in chains of _____.

interneurons

---

243. Interneuronal chains form what has been termed reverberating circuits. These multiple connections cause input to be sustained and amplified and they continue to bombard the efferent neurons even after the stimulus has been removed.

Interneurons may be either excitatory or _____.

inhibitory

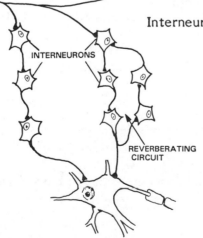

244. It is known that interneurons do not have periods of hyperpolarization as do motor neurons and they are, therefore, capable of _____ activation.

continuous

---

245. The interneuronal cells have the same enhancement properties of monosynaptic transmission such as summation and post-tetanic potentiation.

All these qualities tend to increase and sustain the output of a circuit whether the cells are excitatory or _____.

inhibitory

---

246. It is important to note that the majority of synapses on a motor neuron are with _____.

interneurons

---

247. Ninety-nine percent of the excitatory and inhibitory inputs on motor neurons come from interneurons and from supraspinal influences. Under normal circumstances, the afferent volley from stretch receptors only has a one percent influence on the ultimate motor responses (Davidoff, 1981).

The majority of synapses on a motor neuron are with _____.

interneurons

---

248. Interneurons do not have periods of _____.

hyperpolarization

168

SUMMARY

The Golgi tendon organ (GTO) consists of a connective tissue capsule which contains the ends of a number of extrafusal muscle fibers from a discrete number of motor units. The afferent fiber enters the capsule and gives rise to multiple branches which intertwine with connective tissue bundles from the muscle fibers. Contraction or shortening of the muscle activates the receptor. Thus, the GTO is a tension receptor which is located in the musculotendenous junction.

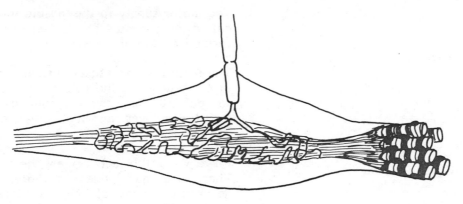

GOLGI TENDON ORGAN

The GTO may be stimulated by passive stretch or active contraction of the muscle. The GTO appears to have a high threshold to passive elongation compared to that of muscle contraction because the joint must be taken to the end of the range of motion to produce much tension. It can, however, monitor the contraction of a single motor unit.

The GTO makes polysynaptic connections with the motor neuron pool. It always produces autogenic inhibition. Muscle spindle effects are primarily localized to the muscle in which they reside whereas the GTO may produce much more widespread effects through its multisynaptic connections.

GTO effects are very strong in extensor muscles and relatively weak in flexor muscles. Very vigorous firing of the GTO occurs in a muscle which is contracting while relatively "fixed" in an elongated position. An example of such a condition is when the soleus muscle is in a relatively lengthened state while contracting during a weight-bearing squat.

It is important to note that the majority of synapses on a motor neuron are with interneurons. Interneuronal cells have many of the same enhancement properties of monosynaptic transmission. These qualities tend to increase or sustain the output of a circuit whether it is excitatory or inhibitory.

249. The intrafusal muscle fibers of the muscle spindle have an efferent or motor nerve supply as do the extrafusal muscle fibers. The motor neuron which supplies the extrafusal muscle fibers is referred to as the alpha motor neuron.

The motor supply to the muscle spindle was originally called the gamma system. More recently, it has been termed the fusimotor system.

The length of extrafusal muscle varies with the state of contraction. The role of the fusimotor system is to permit the muscle spindle to maintain its sensitivity over a wide range of muscle lengths (Kandel, 1981).

First, we will briefly review the alpha motor system. There are many sizes of motor neurons and size determines many of their qualities. There is also evidence that, irrespective of size, there may be other qualities which distinguish types of motor neurons. There are at least three types, one for each of the three _____ fiber types.

muscle

---

250. A large phasic motor neuron will innervate type _____ muscle fibers.

IIA, B (phasic)

---

251. A small tonic motor neuron will innervate type _____ muscle fibers.

I (tonic)

252. Motor units may be classified as type I, IIA and IIB. The largest and fastest (or most phasic) motor unit is a type _____.

IIB

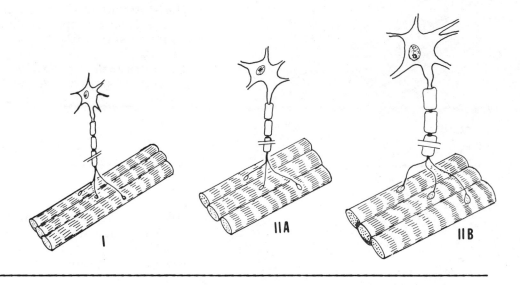

I   IIA   IIB

---

253. The cell body of the alpha motor neuron is called the _____ _____ cell.

anterior horn

---

254. Label the the cell bodies and axons of the phasic and tonic alpha motor neurons.

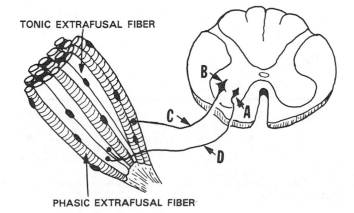

TONIC EXTRAFUSAL FIBER

B

C   A

D

PHASIC EXTRAFUSAL FIBER

A. cell body (tonic)
B. cell body (phasic)
C. axon (tonic)
D. axon (phasic)

255. It may be concluded that there are probably two functional types of intrafusal muscle fibers, just as there are at least two different extrafusal types.

The static nerve fibers generally are thought to come to and from the nuclear chain and static nuclear bag fibers (Ia static, II).

The intrafusal muscle fibers most likely responsible for static functions are the static nuclear bag and the nuclear _____ fibers.

chain

256. The dynamic nuclear bag intrafusal muscle fiber and its innervation are responsible for dynamic functions.

The static intrafusal fibers are the _____ _____ fibers.

nuclear chain and
static nuclear bag

257. The dynamic intrafusal muscle fibers are the _____ _____ _____ fibers.

dynamic nuclear bag

258. The nuclear chain intrafusal muscle fibers most likely are functionally _____.

static

259. The nuclear bag muscle fibers are functionally _____ and _____.

dynamic
static

172

260. The motor supply to the intrafusal muscle fibers (muscle spindle) is referred to as the **fusimotor system.**

For many years this system was thought to be composed entirely of gamma (γ) fibers, and was, therefore, referred to as the gamma system. This is misleading as the muscle spindle is also innervated by beta fibers. The newer terminology for the muscle spindle **efferents** is the fusimotor system.

The fusimotor system is the _____ supply to the _____ _____.

motor or efferent
muscle spindle
or intrafusal muscle

---

261. There has been considerable debate for many years over the anatomy of the fusimotor system. While the debate continues, agreement has been reached on several points. There are probably three types of motor fibers to the muscle spindle. These nerve fibers are called gamma and beta fibers. They have three types of endings: trails, plates, and beta plates.

These fusimotor endings innervate the _____ muscle fibers (Granit, 1970).

intrafusal

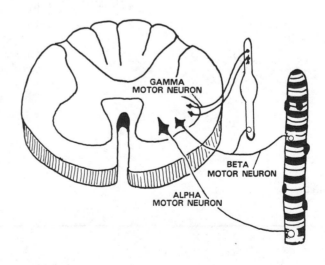

GAMMA
MOTOR NEURON

BETA
MOTOR NEURON

ALPHA
MOTOR NEURON

262. The efferent supply to the muscle spindle is called the _____ system.

fusimotor

---

263. When the contractile elements of an intrafusal muscle fiber shorten, the sensory (equatorial) region is stretched just as if the extrafusal muscle fiber had been stretched.

If the intrafusal muscles contract, the equatorial regions of the muscle fibers are _____.

stretched

---

264. Three types of muscle spindle efferent fiber endings are _____, _____ and beta _____.

trails
plates
plates

---

265. Beta plates are the endings from collaterals of beta fibers. These plates are similar in every respect to extrafusal motor end plates. The literature refers to these beta fibers as alpha fibers of a slower conduction velocity (Granit, 1970).

Therefore, these fibers are often referred to as both alpha fibers and their collaterals, or beta fibers and their collaterals. They are in fact both A fibers. Both nerve fibers terminate in _____ endings.

plate

---

266. Beta fibers are smaller than, but otherwise identical to, _____ fibers.

alpha

174

267. In this volume they will be referred to as beta fibers and beta plates in order to avoid confusion in naming fibers that innervate only extrafusal muscle with those that innervate both intrafusal and extrafusal muscle fibers.

Alpha, beta and gamma fibers are all in the fiber classifications of I and II or _____.

A

---

268. A size fibers of various conduction velocities innervating both intrafusal and extrafusal muscle fibers will be referred to as _____ fibers.

beta

---

269. This beta innervation is sometimes referred to as the skeletofusimotor system because it innervates both _____ and _____ muscle fibers.

intrafusal
extrafusal

---

270. All fusimotor fibers (gamma and beta) have their cell bodies in the ventral horn just as do the _____ motor neurons.

alpha

---

271. II size fibers include a range in size which encompasses both _____ and _____ fibers.

beta
gamma

272. Current evidence indicates that alpha (**α**) motor neurons, beta (**β**) motor neurons and gamma (**ϒ**) motor neurons supplying a given muscle are in close proximity (Bryan, 1972).

The cell bodies of motor neurons are in the ventral horn of the spinal cord. Those alpha, beta and gamma fibers to a specific muscle lie _____ to one another.

close

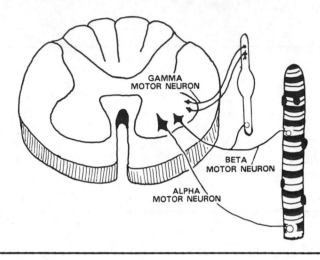

---

273. Within close proximity in the ventral horn of the spinal cord are the motor neurons which innervate a specific muscle. These neurons are the _____ _____ and _____ motor neurons.

alpha (**α**)
beta (**β**)
gamma (**ϒ**)

---

274. Alpha beta, and gamma motor neurons found close together in the ventral horn of the spinal cord innervate a specific _____.

muscle

---

275. If the alpha motor neurons to a specific muscle are arranged in longitudinal columns called motor neuron pools, it stands to reason that the fusimotor neurons are contained within or are closely associated with the _____ _____ _____.

motor neuron pools

276. The fiber ending in a beta (β) plate is a collateral from a beta fiber which also innervates skeletal muscle.

This arrangement probably enhances simultaneous control between intrafusal and _____ muscle fibers.

extrafusal

---

277. Study the diagram.

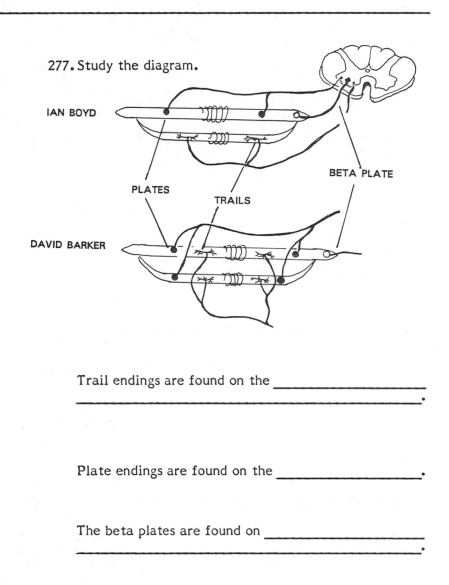

IAN BOYD

PLATES

TRAILS

BETA PLATE

DAVID BARKER

Trail endings are found on the _____.

nuclear chain and static nuclear bag fibers

Plate endings are found on the _____.

dynamic nuclear bag

The beta plates are found on _____.

nuclear bag fibers

177

278. In the following illustration, these symbols will be used for motor endings.

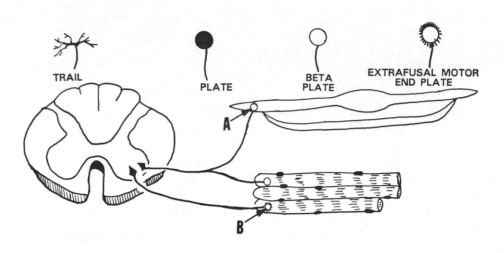

TRAIL   PLATE   BETA PLATE   EXTRAFUSAL MOTOR END PLATE

A is _____
B is _____

A   beta plate
B   extrafusal motor
     end plate

---

279. The fusimotor system maintains the output of the muscle spindle receptors throughout a variety of conditions. If a fusimotor fiber fires it will cause the _____ muscle to _____.

intrafusal
contract

---

280. This system provides an intrinsic motor mechanism for exciting the primary (Ia) and secondary (II) sensory receptors just as these endings are extrinsically excited when extrafusal muscle fibers are _____.

stretched

178

281. The physiological function of the fusimotor system is to provide internal "stretch" to the equatorial region of the intrafusal muscle fibers. This occurs mainly when extrafusal muscle fibers are contracting. The muscle spindle would be unloaded during contraction and be difficult to get firing again were it not for the _____ system.

fusimotor

---

282. A sustained stretch on the extrafusal muscle elongates the muscle spindles, and the static sensory ending fires with a certain frequency.

RECORD FROM
PRIMARY RECEPTOR

EXTRAFUSAL MUSCLE AND
SPINDLE ON STRETCH

OUTPUT FROM
PRIMARY
RECEPTORS

The muscle spindle is stretched when the extrafusal muscle fiber is stretched because they are connected in _____.

parallel

---

283. A maintained stretch to the extrafusal muscle elongates the muscle spindle and results in a sustained output from the _____ sensory endings.

static

284. With experimentation, it has been shown that there is an electrically silent period (recording from the primary sensory fibers) when the extrafusal muscle fibers contract. This means the muscle spindles are so completely "slack" that the sensory fibers will not fire during the twitch.

If, however, the static gamma motor fiber (plate endings--static fusimotor supply) is stimulated during the extrafusal muscle twitch contraction, the afferent fiber continues to fire. (Fig. b)

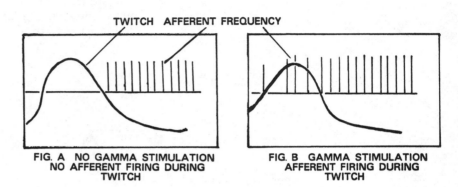

TWITCH   AFFERENT FREQUENCY

FIG. A   NO GAMMA STIMULATION
NO AFFERENT FIRING DURING
TWITCH

FIG. B   GAMMA STIMULATION
AFFERENT FIRING DURING
TWITCH

The static gamma output, therefore, can take up the "_____."

slack

---

285. The equatorial region (receptor site) of the muscle spindle is acted upon by the contracting intrafusal muscle fibers, and the sensory endings are stimulated by this internal _____.

stretch

---

286. The static gamma motor neuron enhances the output or sensitivity of the _____ receptors.

static

287. Fig. a and b (which correspond to electrical tracings of fig. a and b in question 284) illustrate the effect of stimulating the gamma fiber to take up the "slack" at the receptor site of the spindle and permit a sustained discharge even when the extrafusal muscle fibers are _____.

EXTRAFUSAL MUSCLE AND
SPINDLE ON STRETCH

EXTRAFUSAL MUSCLE
CONTRACTION
SPINDLE SLACK

GAMMA STIMULATION
SPINDLE READJUSTS

contracting or
shortening

_____

288. If the muscle spindle is unloaded ("slack") it will take more stretch to stimulate the sensory endings than if it were _____.

taut or stretched

_____

289. The gamma stimulation to the muscle spindle keeps the muscle spindle taut at the receptor site so that it is constantly sensitive to minute changes in muscle _____.

stretch or length

_____

290. Without gamma stimulation, the muscle spindle receptors would be silent during _____ _____ _____.

extrafusal muscle contraction

291. Essentially, the overall function of all components of fusimotor innervation is to keep the muscle spindle sensitive to changes in _____.

length

---

292. The dynamic gamma fibers keep the muscle spindle sensitive **during** changes in extrafusal muscle _____.

length

---

293. When the static gamma system provides background input, the primary receptor (Ia) is more sensitive to a _____ type of stretch.

maintained

---

294. When the dynamic gamma fibers are activated the primary receptor (Ia) is more sensitive to the _____ phase of stretch.

quick
or
phasic

---

295. The secondary receptor (II) is influenced almost exclusively by the _____ gamma motor neurons.

static

296. Label the diagram.

TRAIL

PLATE

BETA
PLATE

EXTRAFUSAL MOTOR
END PLATE

A

B

C

A is _____
B is _____
C is _____

A   gamma trail
B   gamma plate
C   extrafusal motor
     end plate

---

297. Actually, beta plates and extrafusal motor end plates are structurally and functionally _____.

identical

---

298. Gamma plate endings are found mostly on dynamic nuclear bag fibers at the more polar regions of the fiber.

Beta plates are found on both _____ and _____ muscle fibers.

intrafusal
extrafusal

299. The gamma trail endings are found on the nuclear chain and static nuclear bag fibers.

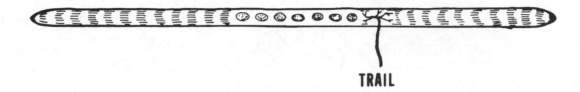

TRAIL

On those fibers the trail endings are located near the _____ region.

equatorial or
non-contractile
or center

---

300. Given the locations and functions of the sensory and motor endings it would appear that the static nuclear bag and nuclear chain fibers are implicated in the length sensitivity of the muscle spindle.

The intrafusal muscle fiber that is most likely implicated in the velocity sensitivity of the muscle spindle is the _____ _____ _____.

dynamic nuclear bag

---

301. Irrespective of the general view that the endings are located as described, there is some evidence that both the plates and trail endings may appear on either fiber.

Plate endings are located on the _____ regions.

polar

302. Label (A through J muscle fibers, and afferent and efferent fibers and indicate static or dynamic where appropriate.

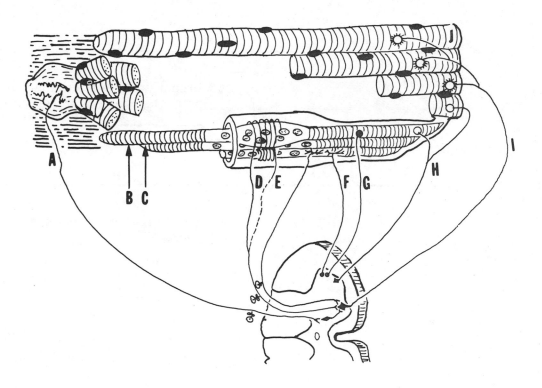

A   GTO
B   Nuclear bag fiber (dynamic)
C   Nuclear chain fiber
D   Primary (Ia) (dynamic component)
E   Primary (Ia) (static component)
F   Gamma trail (static)
G   Gamma plate (dynamic)
H   Beta plate
I   Alpha motor neurons
J   Extrafusal muscle fibers

---

303. The primary fiber sends terminals to most or all of the cells in the _____ _____ pool.

motor neuron

304. The primary afferent inputs, therefore, are found on every motor neuron cell body in the motor neuron pool whether those cells are large or _____.

small

305. Primary afferent terminals are also found on a large percentage of motor neurons to muscles which are _____ of the movement.

synergists

306. The fusimotor system can be put into the functional cycle.

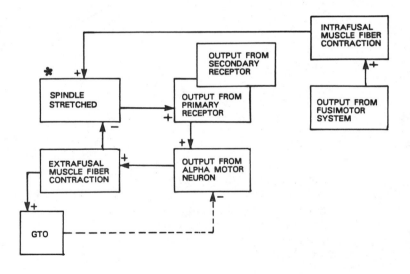

Output from the fusimotor system provides excitation to the _____ _____ _____.

intrafusal muscle fibers

SUMMARY

The motor supply to the extrafusal muscle is the alpha motor neuron.

Beta motor neurons supply both intrafusal and extrafusal muscle fibers. Such a system would provide simultaneous control or co-activation of both types of muscle fibers. Morphologically, beta motor neurons are identical to alpha motor neurons, except that the beta fibers are smaller.

All motor neurons, alpha, beta and gamma, have their cell bodies in the ventral horn. All types of motor neurons which innervate a particular muscle and its muscle spindles lie in close proximity to each other within the ventral horn.

The fusimotor system maintains or enhances the sensitivity of the spindle receptors over a variety of conditions. If a fusimotor fiber fires it will cause the intrafusal muscle to contract. This system provides an intrinsic motor mechanism for exciting primary and secondary sensory receptors by providing internal stretch to the receptor areas in the equatorial region. Activation of the fusimotor system occurs mainly when extrafusal muscle fibers are contracting. Extrafusal contraction unloads the spindle and the spindle would fail to register new muscle lengths if the fusimotor system did not "reset" the sensitivity level.

The dynamic fusimotor fibers which primarily innervate the dynamic nuclear bag fibers (gamma plate endings) keep the muscle spindle sensitive during **changes** in extrafusal muscle length.

The static fusimotor fibers (trail endings) are located primarily on the nuclear chain and static nuclear bag fibers and these static fibers provide background input which keeps the static receptors more sensitive to the maintained length of the extrafusal muscle.

307. To this point it is clear that extrafusal muscle fibers are controlled by the large alpha motor neurons and that the intrafusal fibers are controlled by beta and _____ motor neurons.

gamma

308. In man, there are basically two independent systems in the CNS providing the control over intrafusal and extrafusal muscle. In lower animals there is a simpler system by which only one motor neuron innervates both fibers.

This would correspond to the skeletofusimotor or _____ innervation.

beta

309. The beta system would provide one pathway to activate both intrafusal and extrafusal fibers. On a higher evolutionary scale, however, the dual system predom-inates.

In man, there are two separate systems controlling _____ and _____ muscle fibers.

extrafusal
intrafusal

310. Furthermore, both the static and dynamic fusimotor neurons have somewhat independent control sources as well. For example, the dynamic gamma neurons are influenced more strongly by peripheral input than are the _____ motor neurons (Bishop, 1982).

static gamma

311. Before looking at higher controls, it may be useful to compare the characteristics of gamma motor neurons with those of the alpha system which you already know. Gamma motor neurons are much smaller than the alpha motor neurons with which they are associated.

Remembering the size principle of neuron sensitivity you know that the gamma motor neuron will have a threshold of activation that is _____ than the alpha neuron.

lower

---

312. The after-hyperpolarizations of gamma neurons are of shorter duration than those of the _____ motor neurons.

alpha

---

313. Because the gamma cell size is so small, a single synapse covers a larger part of the total area of the cell body. Thus a single input will have a greater effect on gamma motor neurons than on _____ _____ _____.

alpha motor neurons

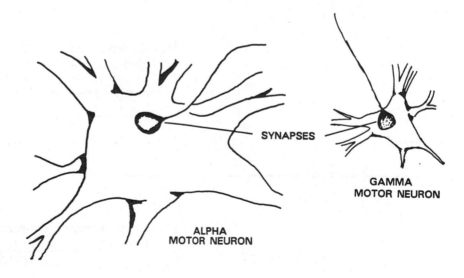

SYNAPSES

GAMMA
MOTOR NEURON

ALPHA
MOTOR NEURON

314. These characteristic differences probably account for the fact that gamma motor neurons are tonically active while, as you remember, alpha motor neurons are not _____ _____.

tonically active

315. Gamma motor neurons do not have monosynaptic excitatory input from their own primary (Ia) fibers. Just as the alpha motor neurons, the gamma neurons do have polysynaptic autogenous inhibitory input from their own _____ (Bishop, 1982).

GTO

316. Gamma motor neurons also receive reciprocal inhibition from primary (Ia) fibers in the antagonist (Bishop, 1982). These connections are not monosynaptic and, therefore, require _____.

interneurons

317. Gamma motor neurons, particularly the dynamic gamma neurons, are excited by cutaneous afferents (Bishop, 1982). Inputs from flexor muscles have a much greater influence than do inputs from _____ muscles.

extensor

318. Gamma motor neurons receive inhibitory input from their own _____ and from the antagonist's _____ receptors.

GTO
Ia

primary receptor (Ia)

319. The gamma motor neurons do not receive excitatory input from their own _____ _____.

_____

cutaneous

320. The dynamic gamma motor neurons receive excitatory input from _____ afferents.

_____

321. Both alpha and gamma motor neurons are controlled by higher centers as well as spinal level mechanisms and peripheral inputs.

You learned earlier that the fusimotor system was active **during** muscle contraction. This means that alpha and gamma motor neurons are being activated simultaneously. This is referred to as alpha-gamma co-activation.

In lower animals this co-activation is accomplished through innervation by the _____ fibers.

beta

_____

322. It is not the purpose of this text to present structure and function underlying higher motor control. The major work presented here is relative to peripheral and spinal control or contributions to movement.

We will, however, briefly list some of the supraspinal mechanisms involved in controlling alpha and gamma motor neurons. The reader is directed to any of the physiology texts listed in the bibliography for further information.

Gamma motor neurons receive autogenous inhibition and reciprocal inhibition from the _____ and _____ receptors, respectively.

GTO (Ib)
primary (Ia)

_____

323. Simultaneous activation of both the extrafusal and intrafusal efferent fibers is referred to as _____ _____.

alpha-gamma co-activation

191

324. Cutaneous input excites dynamic _____ motor neurons.

gamma

---

325. Inputs from flexor muscles have a greater influence on the gamma motor neurons than do those from _____ muscles.

extensor

---

326. Some descending systems that will activate alpha motor neurons will also activate gamma motor neurons. The systems are independent but are believed to be parallel.

Some sites in the brain that can initiate or inhibit movement can activate either the alpha or _____ systems.

gamma

---

327. **Phasic alpha motor neurons.** These cells are activated by corticospinal inputs. Many of these inputs are monosynaptic in nature (Bishop, 1982).

Any activity which strongly recruits phasic motor neurons is driven by _____ inputs.

cortical

---

328. Some areas of the central nervous system provide primary input to one type of motor neuron and not to the others.

The different types of alpha and gamma motor neurons also are affected differently by input from the _____ nervous system.

peripheral

192

329. Tonic alpha motor neurons. One of the most important sources of excitatory input to these cells is from the vestibular system. Many inhibitory projections come from the cerebellum (Bishop, 1982).

Tonic motor units are needed to provide the contractions for postural activities. These are not driven by _____ input.

cortical

---

330. Static gamma motor neurons. These cells are strongly activated by the lateral reticular formation and inhibited by the medial reticular formation. They are controlled by the vestibular system via vestibular input to the reticular formation (Bishop, 1982).

They require supraspinal support and, in comparison to dynamic gamma motor neurons, they are less affected by _____ input.

peripheral

---

331. Dynamic gamma motor neurons. These cells are activated by centers in the tegmentum and inhibited by the cerebellum via the vestibular nuclei. Of the two fusimotor neurons, the dynamic ones are more influenced by _____ input (Bishop, 1982).

peripheral

---

332. Peripheral input includes excitation from cutaneous receptors and receptors located primarily in _____ muscles.

flexor

193

333. There are various modes of inhibitory control over alpha and gamma motor neurons. Some of the higher center inhibitory controls have already been mentioned.

Phasic alpha motor neurons receive inhibitory input from the corticospinal tract via interneurons. Phasic alpha motor neurons also receive their excitatory input from the _____ _____.

corticospinal tract

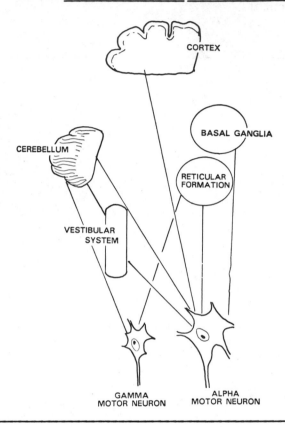

334. Tonic alpha motor neurons receive inhibitory projections via the vestibular nuclei from the _____.

cerebellum

335. Dynamic gamma motor neurons also receive inhibitory projections via the vestibular nuclei from the _____.

cerebellum

336. Static gamma motor neurons are least affected by peripheral input and are inhibited by projections from the medial _____ _____ .

reticular formation

337. All of these motor neurons undoubtedly receive inhibitory projections from other centers in the CNS but those that have been mentioned are the principal ones. It is clear that the different types of neurons receive most of their inputs from different areas of the CNS.

There are various inhibitory mechanisms that occur at the spinal cord level as well. Two of these, which have already been mentioned are autogenous inhibition and reciprocal _____ .

inhibition

338. Another inhibitory system which influences only alpha motor neurons is mediated by specialized interneurons called Renshaw cells. These cells are found only in the ventral horn of the spinal cord.

The Renshaw cells receive a synapse from a branch of the alpha motor neuron. The firing of the alpha motor neuron sends impulses to the Renshaw cell which, in turn, inhibits the alpha motor neuron just fired.

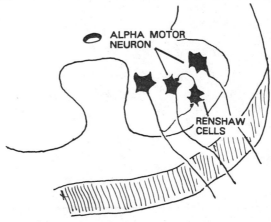

Renshaw cells produce _____ of the alpha motor neuron.

inhibition

195

339. The alpha motor neuron has a branch or collateral which fires on the small interneuronal cells in the ventral part of the spinal cord called _____ cells.

Renshaw

---

340. The Renshaw cells are activated by and in turn act upon the discharging _____ _____ _____.

alpha motor neuron

---

341. Renshaw cells produce what is called **recurrent inhibition.** Renshaw cells, therefore, produce autogenous _____.

inhibition

---

342. The connections made by Renshaw cells are not limited only to the one alpha motor neuron. The Renshaw cell may send branches to other motor neurons in the area. This would produce a more widespread alpha _____.

inhibition

---

343. Renshaw cells mediate _____ inhibition.

recurrent

344. Renshaw cells also terminate in inhibitory synapses on other Renshaw cells and on the interneurons in the primary receptor pathway which mediate reciprocal _____.

inhibition

---

345. Disinhibition will occur if a Renshaw cell receives inhibition from another Renshaw cell. The net effect of inhibiting inhibition is _____.

excitation

---

346. The same mechanism occurs if Renshaw cells produce an inhibiting effect on inhibitory interneurons in a primary afferent pathway. If this inhibition occurs there will be less effect from reciprocal _____.

inhibition

---

347. Renshaw cells are also inhibited by projections from higher centers just as are the _____ and _____ motor neurons.

alpha
gamma

---

348. Renshaw cells receive inputs from a number of sources, however, the greatest influences come from collaterals of the homonymous _____ _____ _____.

alpha motor neurons

197

349. The overall role of the Renshaw system is to suppress repetitive firing of the _____ _____ _____.

alpha motor neuron

350. Renshaw cells also receive excitatory input from the interneurons in the flexor reflex afferent system (FRA's). The FRA system consists of input from various size fibers which when excited produce a net effect of excitation of flexor muscles and inhibition of extensors. None of the largest fibers (A alpha or I) are represented in this group. These fibers come from receptors primarily found in the skin and muscle.

Most likely this FRA input would serve to inhibit extensor motor neurons during a _____ reflex.

flexor

351. It is interesting to note that Renshaw cells are most strongly excited by output from phasic motor neurons, however, phasic motor neurons are very resistant to Renshaw inhibition.

Tonic motor neurons are much more susceptible to _____ _____.

recurrent inhibition

352. The strong resistance of the phasic motor neuron to Renshaw inhibition probably supports the motor neuron's characteristic ability to fire _____.

repetitively

353. So far, we have described the inhibitory effects on alpha motor neurons as:
(1) descending from higher center inhibition,
(2) _____ inhibition,
(3) _____ inhibition, and
(4) _____ inhibition.

autogenous
reciprocal
recurrent

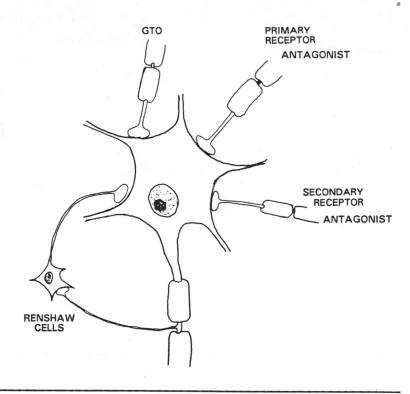

GTO

PRIMARY
RECEPTOR

ANTAGONIST

SECONDARY
RECEPTOR

ANTAGONIST

RENSHAW
CELLS

354. Gamma motor neurons do not receive input from Renshaw cells so they lack _____ inhibition.

recurrent

355. One of the reasons that gamma motor neurons are tonically active and alpha neurons are not may be that the gammas lack _____ _____.

recurrent inhibition

199

356. Another type of inhibition which has widespread effects is pre-synaptic inhibition. This is referred to as primary afferent depolarization or PAD. Pre-synaptic inhibition works through axo-axonic synapses. Through these synapses the effective input from the afferent fiber is reduced before it can excite the motor neurons.

This is why it is called _____ inhibition.

pre-synaptic

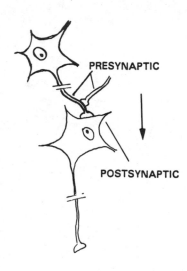

---

357. Pre-synaptic inhibitory effects last 50 to 100 times longer than some forms of post-synaptic inhibition. The selective reduction of excitatory inputs from GTO, primary and cutaneous afferents would serve to reduce the net excitatory effects on _____

motor neurons

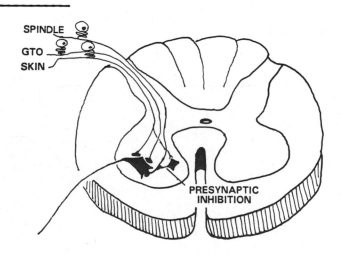

358. The motor neuron which receives the greatest excitation from the primary receptor (Ia) is the _____ _____ motor neuron.

tonic alpha

---

359. Influences on the alpha and gamma motor neurons can be summarized in the following diagram. Fill in the appropriate boxes.

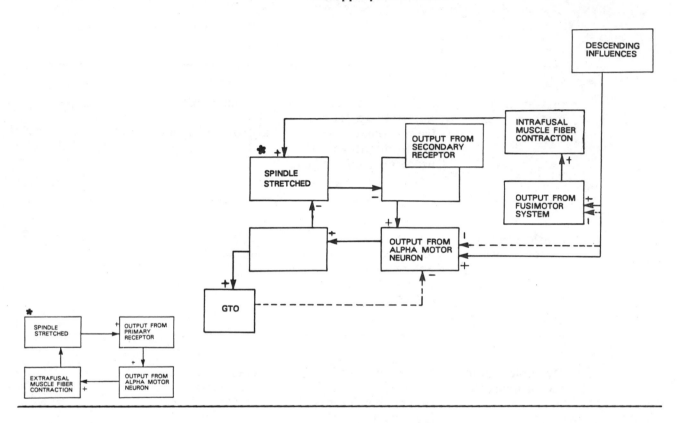

---

360. In this section, we have enumerated some of the excititory and inhibitory influences on alpha and gamma motor neurons. In addition to the differences in input between the two broad classifications of ventral horn motor neurons, there are specific differences within the categories.

The inputs may be different for tonic and phasic alpha motor neurons as well as _____ and _____ gamma motor neurons.

static
dynamic

201

SUMMARY CHART

	Excitatory Influences	Inhibitory Influences
Tonic alpha motor neurons	Vestibular nuclei Primary (Ia) afferent from agonist--high GTO from antagonist	Cerebellum via vestibular nuclei Ia from antagonist GTO Renshaw cells Cutaneous input--high
Phasic alpha motor neurons	Cortical spinal tract Primary (Ia) afferent from agonist--low GTO from antagonist Cutaneous input--high	Renshaw cells GTO Ia from antagonist
Static gamma motor neurons	Lateral reticular formation Require supraspinal support for activation	Medial reticular formation
Dynamic gamma motor neurons	Tegmentum (red nucleus) Cutaneous afferents (particularly from flexors) Joint afferents	Cerebellum via vestibular nuclei

SECTION III

Applied Neurophysiology Relating
to the Muscle Spindle

1. Role of the Stretch Reflexes

2. The Mechanisms in Spasticity

3. Tonic Vibration Reflex

4. Co-Contraction

5. Flexors and Extensors

6. Ranges

ROLE OF THE STRETCH REFLEXES

1. Let us look a little more closely at the function of the muscle spindle afferent and efferent systems. It has been determined that the gamma motor neurons or the fusimotor system provide the "fine tuning" required to keep the spindle responsive to stretch.

   An interesting observation is that primary receptor (Ia) endings are very sensitive to small stretches. During such small stretches the primary afferents are very accurate in their response.

   These responses lose their intensity and accuracy during large changes in muscle _____.

length

2. At the end of large stretches, the receptor can "reset" itself so that in the new range it is once again sensitive to _____ stretches.

small

3. The functional significance of this variability in sensitivity is not clear as most physiologically important movements produce changes in muscle length of a greater magnitude than those to which the primary ending is most sensitive.

   The secondary (II) receptors are less sensitive than primary (Ia) receptors whether the stretch is small or large. The II receptor is, however, much less inconsistent in its responses throughout the range (Mountcastle, 1980).

   The primary receptors are sensitive to _____ stretches.

small

4. The primary sensory endings are not very responsive or accurate when the muscle is undergoing length changes that are _____.

large

5. The secondary receptor more accurately reflects the length of the extrafusal muscle throughout the range than the primary receptor although the secondary ending is less _____ overall.

sensitive

---

6. It is apparent that the CNS is able to make use of these different forms of information. The significance of these differences escapes our understanding at the present. These findings do raise questions as to the function of the muscle spindle output during physiological _____.

movement

---

7. In non-contracting human muscles, primary receptors maintain a steady discharge. Experiments which had included subjects who were performing various maneuvers did not show any change in spindle discharge if the receptor-bearing muscles were not stretched or contracted.

    For example, if the experimenter was recording from spindles in the biceps muscle, moving about without stretching the biceps muscle would not change the primary spindle output. Producing a contraction of the lower extremity muscles also failed to alter spindle output in the biceps muscle.

    The conclusion reached with such experiments is that non-contracting muscles are not subject to fluctuating fusimotor drive which varies when there are changes in mental state or motor preparedness (Burke, 1983).

    These experiments, however, have been conducted on the more superficial distal muscles which normally operate as joint movers. Similar experimentation with deep postural fixating types of muscle are lacking.

    It may not be possible to generalize findings in superficial muscles to the _____ muscles.

deep
or
postural

8. Non-contracting muscles do not exhibit fluctuating fusimotor drive when the individual changes his or her mental _____.

state

---

9. It might be expected that the fusimotor system is more likely to play a significant role when the muscle is _____.

contracting

---

10. Many theories have been postulated as to the role of the muscle spindle in posture and movement. One theory was called the **length-servo** hypothesis. In biological terms, a servomechanism is a feedback system which controls the constancy of activity.

In this theory, the misalignment between intended muscle length and actual muscle length would be determined by activity in the fusimotor system. That is, if the systems were activated by a certain load requirement and the load was increased the gamma output would increase. This would cause the primary endings to increase their output and "drive" the alpha motor neuron. The "drive" would increase muscle contraction to compensate for the load.

With this hypothesis, the contraction of extrafusal muscle would follow automatically the degree of contraction in the _____ muscle.

intrafusal

---

11. Vallbo (1973) showed that spindle acceleration **followed** EMG potentials from contracting muscles rather than preceeding them. It was, therefore, concluded that voluntary contraction is not initiated through the _____ system.

fusimotor

12. Because the discharge frequency of a spindle ending increases as the strength of extrafusal contraction rises, Vallbo concluded that alpha and gamma motor neurons are co-activated.

These experimenters suggested a **servo-assist** mode for load compensation rather than a length-_____ mode.

servo

_____

13. The servo-assistance theory also has been questioned because it is now clear that the supportive excitation available to alpha motor neurons from the spindle loop is not very powerful.

The actual strength of the reflex connections are probably insufficient to play a significant role in _____ compensation.

load

_____

14. The strength of the reflex connections is referred to as the **gain** of the reflex.

The muscle spindle output does not "drive" the alpha motor neuron significantly during contractions because the reflex has an insufficient _____.

gain

_____

15. As the fusimotor outflow closely parallels alpha motor outflow both during contractions and relaxation, this is considered evidence of a tight alpha-gamma "linkage" or co-_____.

activation

_____

16. The strength of the reflex output or response is referred to as the _____ of the reflex.

gain

17. The simplest mechanism for producing such a linkage is the ( ) beta system which links both _____ and _____ muscle.

intrafusal
extrafusal

18. There are both static gamma efferents which are found mostly on nuclear chain and static nuclear bag fibers, and the dynamic gamma fibers which innervate nuclear bag fibers. The effects on spindle endings would be to increase _____ sensitivity for the former and the _____ sensitivity for the latter.

static
dynamic

19. Beta fibers predominate in lower animals but have also been found to be quite extensive in the cat. The extent of the beta system in man is not known, however, there is no question that in man the gamma portion of the fusimotor system is dominant.

The major advantage of such a system in which the output to the intrafusal muscles is separate from the output to intrafusal muscles appears to be the resultant flexibility in alpha-gamma linkage.

This flexibility would not be possible with a predominately _____ system.

beta

20. As noted before, there is little if any spindle afferent excitatory feedback onto gamma motor-neurons. The excitatory feedback is present only on the alpha motor neurons. Therefore, one way to alter alpha-gamma balance from peripheral input is through activity in the stretch reflex such as with muscle contraction.

If the spindle is activated the feedback will go to the alpha motor neurons rather than gamma motor neurons. Therefore, stretch reflex activity will shift the emphasis on the alpha-gamma linkage in favor of the _____ motor neurons.

alpha

21. Because different descending systems have different effects on motor neuron pools, it is quite likely that volitional activation of corticospinal activated muscles such as the small muscles of the hand will produce a different alpha-gamma balance than more sub-cortically activated postural type muscles.

If a muscle changes roles from a prime-mover to a fixator there may be also a change in _____ balance.

alpha-gamma

---

22. When vestibulospinal and reticulospinal pathways are activated by irrigating the ear with warm water there is a lowering of the threshold of spindle afferents (Burke, 1980).

Because the spindle threshold is determined by the amount of fusimotor activity, it is clear that such vestibulospinal and reticulospinal inputs shift the linkage in favor of the _____ neurons.

fusimotor

---

23. Vibration applied to the **skin** of the dorsum of the foot during a voluntary contraction lowered the threshold for spindle activation (Burke, 1980).

Vibration applied to certain regions of the plantar surface raised spindle thresholds.

Thus cutaneous input from certain mechanoreceptors can change the balance depending upon the _____ vibrated.

area

---

24. Cortically activated muscles which produce fine movement such as the intrinsic muscles of the hand will most likely produce a different shift in the alpha-gamma linkage than will a sub-cortically controlled _____ muscle.

postural

25. Although the co-activation of alpha and gamma motor neurons is an important aspect of motor organization, it is clear that alpha, dynamic gamma and static gamma motor neurons can be controlled by centers in the CNS which are independent of one another.

It seems that there is flexibility in alpha-gamma linkage and that descending inputs, stretch reflex changes and other peripheral inputs may modify this _____.

balance or linkage

26. We can hypothesize about the relationship of the alpha-gamma linkage to movement.

If the gamma system provides reflex support for muscle contraction, it would appear that a close linkage would be important. In lower animals this linkage would be "built-in" by the beta innervation. In this situation the linkage would also be very stereotyped and inflexible.

In man, the flexibility of moving to a greater predominance of either gamma or alpha output could provide a base for wide _____ in movement.

variation

27. The ability to utilize a repertoire of alpha-gamma linkages most likely permits man to produce a wide variation in movement and perhaps a greater adaptability to stimuli than _____ animals.

lower

28. Since the alpha and gamma systems are controlled by independent but parallel centers, we might expect lesions in different areas of the CNS to induce different outcomes.

A lesion in an area which controls the gamma motor neurons should either increase or decrease the level or quality of control over the _____ neurons.

gamma

211

29. The term "load dependent assistance" was utilized to describe the function of the stretch reflex as a result of studies done during voluntary shortening contractions.

If the sole function of the fusimotor system is to detect an error in muscle length then there should be no spindle activity if there are no performance errors.

Muscle spindle recordings showed a greater fusimotor drive and a greater spindle output when the ankle dorsiflexors were required to work against a load during a dorsiflexion movement. When exactly the same movement was performed without a load there was an insignificant discharge from spindle endings. Since the movement was the same in both cases, no muscle length error should have occurred. And yet, the spindle output changed because the load changed (Burke, et.al., 1978).

In these studies it was found that spindle activity during a shortening movement depends on the size of the external load. In the experiments, the joints continued through the same arc of movement. Thus, there were no errors in performance; only the loads were changed during the movements.

A more accurate hypothesis of stretch reflex function may be the "_____ dependent servo _____" hypothesis.

load
assistance

---

30. Spindle activity during a shortening movement depends on the size of the external _____.

load

---

31. Evidence indicates that it is not the sole function of the fusimotor system to detect errors in muscle _____.

length

32. If the speed of movement is increased, it becomes increasingly difficult for spindle endings to maintain their discharge.

Some investigators (Prochazka, et.al., 1979) have calculated that if the speed of muscle shortening exceeds a certain rate, fusimotor activity is less dominant than it is at lower speeds of shortening.

These findings show a decrease in the effectiveness of co-activation of alpha and _____ drive.

gamma

---

33. It is apparent that free rapid cyclical movements will receive very little support through stretch reflex pathways. Any fusimotor activity is probably ineffective and irrelevant to such movements. That is, in fast movements it is doubtful that the alpha motor neurons receive enough input from the muscle spindle system to add enough excitation to assist in the movement (Burke, 1983).

Slow movements, especially those which are performed against a load, may require or receive some degree of reflex support.

Thus, we can see that even the "load-dependent servo assistance hypothesis" is only true for certain types of movement.

Stretch reflex support is not required in _____ movements.

fast

---

34. Stretch reflex pathways of the muscle spindle system may provide some reflex support or strength during _____ movements.

slow

---

35. There is a decrease in effectiveness of alpha-gamma co-activation during _____ movements.

rapid
or
fast

213

36. One way in which the muscle spindles could influence movement is that they could encode unwanted changes in acceleration during smooth movements by decreasing output as the speed increases. The resultant lack of any spindle support may decrease some alpha activity and thereby slow or decrease extrafusal muscle _____ (Burke, 1983).

contraction

---

37. Experimentors have further altered the servo-assistance hypothesis based on the timing of reflex responses. An EMG response to stretch or disturbances have been measured at 60 msec. This response delay is too long to be the result of monosynaptic circuits. It is also too short to be considered a voluntary response.

These findings suggest that reflex compensation for changes in load require the involvement of centers or pathways higher than the spinal cord (Marsden, 1973; Evarts, 1973). These responses show that monosynaptic circuits would not be adequate for the load compensation. Some experimentors have called this the transcortico servo-assistance loop. Others have postulated that the reflex response to load compensation involves long latencies through multiple loops and circuits in sub-cortical centers (Crago, et.al., 1976).

Some stretch reflex responses appear to require the involvement of _____ _____.

higher centers

---

38. The role of the stretch reflex at the spinal or segmental level may be to regulate muscle stiffness (Kandel, 1981). The state of stiffness or compliance of the muscle would affect the resistance to disturbance of the limb. This regulation requires information about muscle tension as well as muscle length.

Muscle stiffness could be regulated by the interaction of the _____ _____ and the _____.

muscle spindle
GTO

214

39. It may be misleading to be overly concerned with the idea of **strength** or "gain" of reflex assistance. Movement changes can occur through the increased firing rate of active motor neurons. Changes in movement can also occur because the pattern of active motor units is altered.

For example, if we give each motor unit a number such as 1, 2, 3 and so forth, and assume that units 4, 5 and 10 are active, the movement may be different than if units 1, 3 and 7 are active.

Error correction in movement programs through reflex activity most likely would result in subtle adjustments to the firing patterns of active motor neurons, rather than changes in total muscle power. The latter would occur with changes in the discharge rates of active motor units, especially large ones (Burke, 1983).

Ordinary movement most likely does not require strong _____ assistance.

reflex

Error correction most likely involves a subtle activation of different motor units rather than an increase in the output of the _____ motor unit.

same

---

40. Voluntary contractions are not initiated or maintained by muscle spindle activity. A reflex contraction, on the other hand, is a result of a change in afferent activity.

The muscle spindle provides the afferent input for the stretch reflex. The response of these endings can be changed by fusimotor input.

Because of these relationships, the fusimotor system has often been labeled as the mechanism which controls the gain of the _____ reflex.

stretch

215

41. The fusimotor system was hypothesized to be the mechanism which controls the gain of the stretch reflex. This appeared to be logical reasoning since the increased output of the fusimotor system should increase the output frequency of the afferent fibers.

Increased afferent output was thought to be sufficient to drive the alpha motor neuron.

The alpha output increases the state of muscle contraction, therefore, it would appear logical to assume that increased fusimotor drive was responsible for stretch reflex _____.

gain

---

42. It is difficult to study stretch reflexes in the relaxed human. Only the tendon jerk can be demonstrated and it probably has no useful relationship to normal movement.

When human muscles are not contracting, there is little _____ drive.

fusimotor

---

43. When muscles are contracting, however, there is an increase in fusimotor drive to the spindles in those muscles.

It has been demonstrated then that voluntary contractions will change the gain of _____ reflex pathways.

stretch

---

44. The change in reflex gain is apparent during voluntary contraction. The question is whether the gain change is the result of alteration in fusimotor drive.

One would expect an increase in fusimotor drive to sensitize the spindle endings, causing a greater output. This output would cause a change in the excitability of the alpha motor neurons.

The net result of this chain would be a change in the reflex _____.

gain

216

45. A different consideration is that the reflex gain may occur centrally through a change in reflex transmission.

Any change in the central excitability that would alter the output to alpha motor neurons could be independent of the _____ system.

fusimotor

---

46. Because the earliest change in spindle activity during voluntary contractions **follows** the onset of contraction, these changes have to occur through some mechanism other than the _____ system.

fusimotor

---

47. When an abrupt stretch is applied to a contracting muscle by perturbation of joint position, the muscle produces a burst of reflex activity. It is fair to say that the gain of the reflex has been increased.

The muscle spindle response, however, was no larger than that found when perturbations were produced to a non-contracting muscle. In this latter case a much smaller reflex contraction of the extrafusal muscle occurred.

The increase of the gain in the stretch reflex response in the muscle occurred when comparing contracting versus non-contracting muscle in spite of the same spindle response in both cases (Burke, et.al., 1978).

It is fair to say, then, that this change in reflex gain may be independent of the _____ system.

fusimotor

---

48. Experiments with the tonic vibration reflex show that the reflex can be supressed voluntarily without associated reduction in muscle spindle activity.

The ability to effect some voluntary control over the reflex gain in this instance is mediated through a central mechanism which does not involve the _____ system.

fusimotor

49. Some recent physiological evidence shows that the fusimotor drive is not responsible for the gain of the _____ reflex (Burke, 1983).

stretch

---

50. It was noted that reflex gain may increase following a perturbation to either a contracting or non-contracting muscle.

It was concluded that this change was independent of fusimotor activity because there was no change in the output of the _____ _____.

muscle spindle

---

51. The gain of stretch reflex pathways is apparently a function of some central mechanism rather than the _____ _____.

fusimotor system

---

52. The muscle spindle contibution to stretch reflexes and to functional movement is difficult to assess. It is becoming clear that spindle output is not strong enough to drive alpha motor output. In slow, resisted contraction, however, it most likely does supply some reflex support or assistance to the muscle contraction.

Rapid, cyclical movements probably receive little assistance through _____ _____ pathways.

stretch reflex

---

53. Whatever the function of the fusimotor system may be, it does not appear to be responsible for enhancing stretch reflex _____.

gain

54. Most importantly, when considering the functional roles of the muscle spindle, it should be remembered that the muscle spindle is a sense organ. It projects to the higher centers in the nervous system and even likely to the cortex for conscious awareness.

It is probable that input at this higher level is far more important in a complex motor program than it is at the spinal level reflex mechanism.

It is apparent that muscle spindle input is not necessary for the ability to move or to sense movement and position if other sensory systems (visual, tactile, labyrinthine, other proprioceptors) are intact.

The most important role of the muscle spindle may be to provide _____ to higher centers.

feedback or information

---

55. Our more recent understanding of the role of the muscle spindle in movement does not mean that the knowledge of muscle spindle physiology will be useless in patient treatment.

The contribution of the muscle spindle is probably subtle. The CNS integrates this output along with other sources of information. In reality, it is likely to be just another one of our sensory systems which provide feedback to the CNS and which may on occasion provide some reflex support for _____.

movement

---

56. Patients afflicted with disorders of motor control should greatly benefit from therapeutic intervention if treatment is based on careful observation of the patient's response.

Muscle spindle feedback would be particularly important if there are deficits in other _____ mechanisms.

sensory

57. A major role of the muscle spindle may be in motor learning. When someone learns a new motor task, the movements are usually slow and small.

These conditions are the most likely ones for which co-activated fusimotor drive could produce an appropriate stimulus to the spindle afferents in the contracting muscle. This spindle discharge could provide sensory feedback information to the CNS to develop the motor plan (Burke, 1983).

When a movement skill can be done rapidly and without thinking about it, reflex assistance is probably _____.

unnecessary

---

58. Feedback from the muscle spindle may be most beneficial in retraining or learning new motor tasks.

Repetition of an appropriate activity would provide a "feel" for the _____ movement.

correct
or
desired

---

59. Earlier in this book it was noted that the dynamic primary (Ia) receptor could be stimulated, thus facilitating its own muscle, by a **fast mechanical stretch** of the muscle in which the muscle spindle is located.

The static primary (Ia) receptor may be stimulated by **sustained** or **maintained mechanical stretch** of the muscle in which it is located.

The secondary (II) receptor is also fired by **maintained mechanical stretch** and produces its greatest effect near the physiological limits of the muscle at the end of joint range.

The primary (Ia) dynamic receptor is fired by _____ mechanical stretch and primary (Ia) static and secondary (II) receptors are stimulated by _____ mechanical stretch.

quick
maintained

60. The fusimotor system will provide a second way to produce a stretch stimulus to the muscle spindle. The system produces contraction of the muscle spindle fibers themselves. Such activity provides an **internal** stretch to the spindle afferents.

This system is activated by **maintained contraction** of the extrafusal muscle fibers. The first method, mentioned previously, was mechanical stretch to the extrafusal muscle fibers.

The two ways of stimulating the muscle spindle are _____ _____ and maintained _____ _____.

mechanical stretch
muscle contraction

---

61. A maintained **contraction** of the extrafusal muscle fibers (usually done against maintained resistance) will activate both _____ and _____ receptors.

primary (Ia)
secondary (II)

---

62. Such maintained resistance drives the fusimotor system, which in turn supports the drive of the alpha motor system. As a result the extrafusal muscle produces a _____ contraction.

maintained

---

63. The cycle continues to repeat itself as long as resistance is _____.

maintained

64. The stronger the muscle contraction the greater will be the _____ drive.

fusimotor

---

65. The muscle spindle support for muscle contraction is probably limited to slow, maintained contractions within a narrow range of motion, particularly when _____ is added.

resistance

---

66. Rapid movements probably do not involve muscle _____ support.

spindle

---

67. If your patient is performing slow maintained, resisted contractions he will receive some muscle spindle reflex support. Probably just as important, or even more importantly, he will be sending proprioceptive information to his _____ _____.

higher centers

---

68. The fusimotor system is a mechanism which provides **internal** stretch to a muscle as opposed to external _____ stretch.

mechanical

222

69. To utilize the reflex support for alpha motor neuron activation in your patient, you will want to concentrate on slow _____ _____ .

maintained muscle contractions with resistance added to further enhance the result.

---

70. During eccentric or lengthening contractions the muscle spindle responses are greater than they are to passive stretch of similar amplitude and velocity (Burke, et.al., 1978).

This response suggests that fusimotor activity is heightened during _____ contractions.

eccentric or lengthening

---

71. By convention, physiologists refer to all anti-gravity muscles as "extensors" and to their antagonists as "_____."

flexors

---

72. Stretch reflexes are present in all muscles but are most highly developed in anti-gravity muscles. In animals all antigravity muscles are extensors. These muscle groups are called, therefore, physiological extensors (Mountcastle, 1980; Kandel, 1981).

In man the physiological extensors of the lower extremity are extensor muscles. In the upper extremity the antigravity muscles are _____ muscles

flexor

73. Antigravity muscles (physiological extensors) show maintained reflex contraction to maintained stretch. That is, the contraction lasts as long as the stretch lasts (Mountcastle, 1980).

In general, flexor muscles respond to an abrupt stretch with a brief contraction. Physiological flexors do not usually exhibit a _____ contraction.

maintained

---

74. The muscles that usually exhibit the strongest phasic stretch reflexes are the physiological _____.

flexors

---

75. The muscles which usually demonstrate a maintained contraction as long as the stretch persists are the physiological _____.

extensors

---

76. Physiological extensors are the _____ muscles.

anti-gravity

---

77. The stretch reflexes are best developed in the muscle that was stretched as opposed to its _____.

synergists

SUMMARY

Experiments on distal superficial muscles which are not contracting show that the muscle spindle's output does not fluctuate with mental activities or motor preparedness if the muscle itself is not stretched or contracting.

Several theories have been postulated as to the role of the muscle spindle in posture and movement. Most of them have been discounted. The stretch reflex supports muscle contraction only in slow movements and particularly when resistance is added. Stretch reflexes do not appear to participate in large, rapid, cyclical movements.

The fusimotor outflow closely parallels alpha motor outflow. This activity is referred to as alpha-gamma linkage. Two separate systems for controlling the intrafusal and extrafusal muscles allows considerable flexibility in this linkage. Flexibility in the linkage probably contributes to man's ability to produce a great variety of movements in response to sensory stimuli or voluntary desire.

Stretch reflex activity and certain cutaneous inputs shift the alpha-gamma linkage in favor of the alpha motor system. Vestibulospinal and reticulospinal pathways shift the linkage in favor of the gamma motor neurons.

The **gain** of the stretch reflex can be augmented by voluntary muscle contractions and other mechanisms. This gain may occur centrally and is independent of the fusimotor system.

When considering the functional roles of the muscle spindle it should be remembered that the muscle spindle is a sense organ. Its most important role may be to provide feedback or information to higher centers.

One of the aims of patient treatment should be to provide normal sensory feedback to areas of the nervous system which have been receiving abnormal feedback. Guiding patients through normal movements should help provide this necessary feedback.

78. A clear definition of spasticity escapes us despite the fact that therapists can invariably recognize its presence. Among other things, it has been considered to be a state of hyperexcitability or an increase in the passive resistance to stretch.

Perhaps more useful is a list which characterizes some of the motor signs of spasticity (Nathan, 1963; Bishop, 1971).

1. normally latent stretch reflexes appear

2. phasic stretch reflexes such as the tendon jerk have a lower threshold of activation

3. the tapped muscle produces a greater than normal response

4. synergists may also contract (the stretch reflex is normally very localized to the muscle stretched)

5. tonic stretch reflexes are also enhanced so that resistance to passive movement is apparent

6. clonus may be elicited

Spasticity is the result of numerous alterations in the input controls to the _____.

muscle
or
alpha motor neuron

---

79. It is not useful to describe spasticity as an alteration in muscle "tone." Measurements and definitions of this "tone" have been elusive despite much effort by researchers.

Spasticity is sometimes defined as a resistance to passive stretch. Perhaps the most useful approach at this time is to consider the symptoms or _____ signs of spasticity.

motor

80. The classical views of spasticity and rigidity have come from animal experiments. As time passes it is becoming more and more clear that these models and their classical explanations are not sufficient.

The classical view of spasticity is that a spinal or cerebral lesion **releases** the stretch reflexes from the normal inhibitory mechanisms that control them.

This view is called the _____ phenomenon.

release

---

81. Suppose A controls B and B controls C which in turn influences A.

If a lesion occurs at C, then the influences it once exerted over A are **released.** It is the uncontrolled activity of A which produces many of the symptoms that may be encountered.

This sequence is termed a _____ _____.

release phenomenon

---

82. The corticospinal tract provides excitation to the alpha motor neurons. When a lesion is limited to this tract a flaccid paralysis results. This effect tells us that the corticospinal neurons are not responsible for major inhibitory input to the _____ _____.

motor neurons

227

83. Descending inhibitory input is carried by descending pathways other than the corticospinal tract. If certain areas of this system are injured there is a loss of inhibition, thus it has been concluded that the support for rigidity comes from the _____ tracts.

descending

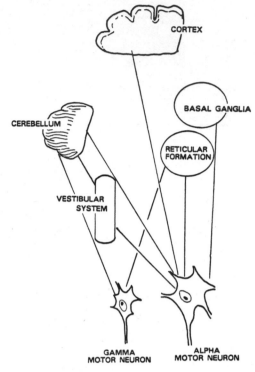

84. Under normal conditions, the inhibitory or supressor areas of the brain balance the excitatory impulses which are generated. Those inhibitory areas include the basal ganglia and areas of the cerebellum and the cortex.

Research suggests that fibers which project from those areas do not end directly on motor neurons but rather terminate in the medial reticular formation. The medial reticular formation cells are diffusely dispersed in the brain stem. They are not "self-driving" and are, therefore, inactive if not driven by input from the supressor areas.

The descending fibers of the medial reticular formation do synapse in the spinal cord and produce the _____ inputs at that level.

inhibitory

inhibition

85. If any of the inhibitory centers are damaged, the result would be that the motor neurons would have less _____.

86. There are specific areas in the nervous system which function to inhibit or suppress neurons in other areas. These are called suppressor areas. The suppressor areas also inhibit excitatory centers as well as excite neurons in the medial reticular formation. The vestibular nuclei, for example, facilitate alpha and gamma motor neurons and are ordinarily suppressed or modified by a suppressor area.

If its supressor area is damaged the vestibular mechanism will go unchecked and produce excessive _____.

facilitation
or
excitation

87. There are specific higher centers in the nervous system which exclusively or primarily produce inhibitory relays. In the discussion of the control of motor neurons you encountered some of the known pathways which specifically act upon the particular types of alpha and gamma motor neurons.

Consider the two major descending motor pathways. Experimental evidence indicates that a "pure" lesion of the corticospinal tract does not contribute to rigidity or _____.

spasiticity

88. Spasticity will not occur with a so-called pure lesion of the _____ tract.

cortico-spinal

89. The classical experiments seemed to indicate that the lack of supression from descending tracts resulted in either excessive input to the alpha neurons (alpha rigidity) or to the gamma motor neurons (_____ rigidity).

gamma

---

90. Following through with logical reasoning based on muscle spindle physiology the role of the fusimotor system in spasticity was hypothesized.

One might expect that if the gamma motor neuron receives excessive input, these neurons would produce an excessive fusimotor drive. Excessive fusimotor drive will produce an increased output from the muscle spindle afferents. Increased spindle output would, therefore, result in excessive drive on the alpha motor neurons.

The end result of such a cycle would appear to be an increased state of muscle contraction and early physiologists considered this cycle to be the cause of _____.

spasticity

---

91. It has also been assumed that spinal level inhibitory mechanisms such as autogenic and recurrent inhibition are not of sufficient strength to compensate for the loss of supraspinal _____ mechanisms.

inhibitory

---

92. Whether the input is directly facilitating alpha motor neurons or indirectly facilitating them through the gamma motor neurons, this excessive activity could be the result of a _____ phenomenon.

release

93. You will remember that under normal circumstances the strength of stretch reflex support is not adequate to normally, let alone excessively, drive _____ motor neurons.

alpha

---

94. In fact, it is now apparent that the so-called release phenomenon which removes tonic inhibitory inputs to alpha and gamma motor neurons at best contributes only a small part to the explanation for _____.

spasticity

---

95. One of the most important topics for us to explore as therapists is the concept of excessive fusimotor drive in spasticity. According to the older view, this drive would result in excessively sensitive primary afferents. Thus any stretch to a spastic muscle would "drive" the alpha motor neuron resulting in even greater extrafusal muscle _____.

contraction

---

96. Work done by Burke and others (1978, 1979, 1982) strongly indicates that there is no excessive fusimotor drive in disorders of muscle "tone".

According to Burke's research and his critical review of the literature (Burke, 1983) there is no evidence to conclude that there is excessive discharge of primary endings in spasticity.

Earlier we noted that the fusimotor system was not responsible for setting the "gain" of _____ reflexes.

stretch

231

97. It was also noted that the strength of stretch reflex input is not sufficient to "drive" the extrafusal _____.

muscle

---

98. Rather, stretch reflexes **assist** in sustaining extra-fusal contraction if the movement is small and slow, and if _____ is added.

resistance

---

99. It is possible that some defect in fusimotor function exists in spasticity, however, there is no irrefutable evidence that there is **excessive** _____ output.

fusimotor

---

100. Does this mean that spasticity and rigidity are the figments of some clinician's imagination? Is it your imagination that the application of stretch to a spastic muscle increases the resistance in that muscle? Absolutely not!

Even carefully controlled experiments show that in spasticity there is an increased stretch reflex upon passive movement (Sahrmann and Norton, 1977).

It is evident, however, that the defect probably lies somewhere in the central mechanisms of the spinal cord, not in the muscle spindle system. Most likely, this would be a change in the outflow from the interneuron _____.

pool

101. The mechanism by which the proprioceptive reflexes such as the stretch reflexes are magnified or potentiated is most likely through changes in the _____ _____.

interneuron pool

---

102. Recent studies suggest that there may be defects in recurrent inhibition and possibly pre-synaptic inhibitory mechanisms in spasticity.

Such defects may result from altered input to the _____ pool.

interneuron

---

103. In the presence of spasticity the muscle spindle is not in itself hyperactive. Rather, the outflow to alpha motor neurons from central mechanisms is _____.

excessive

---

104. As we noted before, in the normal individual the stretch reflex gain increases as the level of voluntary contraction increases (Nielson, 1972a, b).

This response is probably modulated by long latency or long loop reflexes. That is, the level of gain is controlled by supraspinal structures and mediated via the _____ pool.

interneuron

105. In spastic patients there is no further increase in reflex gain even if the muscle contraction is increased. The stretch reflex in these patients is "switched" on and maintained at a high level (Burke, et.al., 1978). This is most likely the result of a loss of modulating effects in the long loop reflexes.

The stretch reflex gain is hyperactive because of loss of the _____ _____ reflexes.

long loop

---

106. Thus, when a spastic muscle is stretched the ordinary extra input from the muscle spindle is added to the already heightened excitability state of central circuits.

The net effect is increased resistance to passive _____.

stretch

---

107. Sahrmann and co-workers (1974, 1977) have further elucidated the movement defects in spasticity. It is clear that the patient's inability to perform voluntary, rapid, repetitive movements has no relationship to the stretching of the antagonist during these movements.

Rather the patient cannot "shut off" the contraction of the spastic muscle at the end of the previous movement cycle.

In spastic patients there is prolonged activity when the muscle should be in a relaxation phase. This continued contraction is most likely maintained by continued reverberations within the _____ circuits.

interneuron

108. When a normal individual performs rapid flexion and extension of the elbow, there is a cessation of the flexor activity at the peak of flexion.

In the spastic patient flexor activity persists throughout the flexion phase and even into the _____ phase.

extension

---

109. The inability of the spastic patient to move rapidly is not the result of stretch reflexes in the antagonistic muscle groups.

Rapid movement requires the ability to generate appropriate tension and _____ .

shut it off
or
release it

---

110. Thus, the excessive response from the tendon tap is a good indication of the central state within the spinal cord but is not a measure of the sensitivity of the _____ _____ .

muscle spindle

---

111. Recent evidence is beginning to clarify some of the questions about spasticity, although much remains to be known.

The first errors made were most likely in assuming that the **acute** condition in the decerebrate cat bears any true resemblance to the **chronic** development of spasticity in man (Burke, 1983). In man, the changes in resistance to passive movement are usually slow to develop.

In fact, a lesion in the CNS produces a whole series of secondary changes at many different levels. These changes occur along a time continuum which begins in seconds and continues for hours, days, weeks, months, and even _____ (Bishop, 1982).

years

112. We know from recent studies that one neuron has a direct effect upon any other neuron upon which it synapses. Death or injury to one neuron has widespread effects on associated neurons resulting ultimately in a variety of reactions, including structural alterations (Bishop, 1982).

Because these alterations of structure have been observed it has become clear that the nervous system does indeed have regenerative and growth capabilities which in the past have been considered unlikely to occur. These findings attest to the plasticity of the CNS.

A CNS lesion results in an array of **dynamic** responses which include alterations in both _____ and function.

structure

---

113. CNS plasticity includes an array of _____ responses.

dynamic

---

114. Death or injury to one neuron has widespread effects on _____ _____.

associated neurons

---

115. If a peripheral motor neuron is injured by transection of its axons many profound effects occur in both the motor neuron and the muscle fiber which it supplies. These effects will not be enumerated here. Our attention concerns the pre-synaptic boutons of fibers **terminating** on the motor neuron.

The monosynaptic input from these boutons is lost or altered as the boutons are displaced from the cell. If the neuron regenerates the lost synaptic input is restored.

Death or injury to one cell results in changes to those cells which _____.

are associated
with it

116. Some changes noted after sectioning the spinal cord are synaptic reclamation by collateral sprouting of surviving neurons which innervate the same structure, and denervation hypersensitivity.

Terminals of spinal interneurons involved in polysynaptic spinal reflexes are called "C" terminals. With certain lesions, these increase in number and size and change shape and location (Bishop, 1982).

These examples of synaptic reorganization in the spinal cord undoubtedly contribute to the abnormalities of motor control and muscle "tone" in spinal lesions.

These responses also help to explain why secondary changes in neuronal function may continue for a relatively long period of _____.

time

---

117. An incoming afferent fiber branches and makes contact with many cells over many spinal segments. Functionally, however, it appears that the receptive field is very discrete and localized.

Recent studies suggest that most of these multiple synapses are ineffective. If a dorsal root is cut, however, these synapses become effective and are no longer dormant (Bishop, 1982).

Apparently the CNS has many more synaptic connections than are necessary for normal _____.

function

---

118. Many synapses in the nervous system appear to be dormant. These connections are made during development but are not usually activated.

When certain lesions occur these dormant synapses become _____.

active

119. Most of the adaptive changes found in the periphery and in the spinal cord are probably also present in the brain. The result may be that afferent synapses that are lost from one source become occupied by synapses from another source.

Thus the CNS may make use of previously unused pathways or establish new pathways during recovery from _____.

lesions or
insults

---

120. Some of the dynamic responses of the nervous system to injury, or what has been termed CNS plasticity, may be to make use of previously unused pathways or to establish _____ _____.

new pathways

---

121. It is not necessarily true that the new pathways result in activity that actually **enhances** function. In fact, the new pathways may be _____ to function.

detrimental

---

122. Collateral sprouting, activating inactive synapses, and reinnervation by previouisly unrelated structures are a few examples of possible short and long term changes in the CNS in response to injury. These are the changes that most likely result in altered function such as spasticity.

This evidence of plasticity in the CNS also suggests that treatment prognosis might be changed as new information surfaces.

Clearly, time will be a factor both in promoting and preventing certain responses during recovery through the treatment program.

If time is of importance then it would be wise to begin treatment programs _____.

early

123. Early treatment intervention might limit some of the unwanted CNS changes by not allowing continuous influences to occur over a long _____.

time

---

124. In view of the unabating nature of some influences, another consideration should be the length of the treatment "session" itself.

If the influences continue 24 hours a day, treatment intervention may be necessary _____ a day.

24 hours

---

125. The synapses which are involved in spasticity are subjected to overuse through prolonged repetitive activity. We already know from the study of post-tetonic potentiation that synapses will alter their efficency of activity when such use is maintained.

Alteration in synaptic efficiency results in the presence of prolonged _____ _____.

repetitive activity

---

126. The transmitting power of a synapse is increased following a period of intense activity. This increase is referred to as _____ _____.

post-tetanic potentiation

---

127. The effects of post-tetanic potentiation (PTP) may persist for a _____ time.

long

The motor units which are most susceptible to PTP are the type _____ units.

I (SO, S)

128. There is apparently type I muscle fiber hypertrophy in spasticity and type I atrophy in flaccidity, at least in stroke patients (Castle, et.al., 1979).

In general, it seems that type I atrophy occurs when there is prolonged decrease in tonic contractions and hypertrophy occurs when there is prolonged _____ in tonic contractions.

increase

---

129. Interesting results have been found from muscle biopsies performed on children with spastic cerebral palsey who had multiple contractures and who were under anesthesia for surgical procedures (Castle, et.al., 1979).

By moving their joints while the children were under anesthesia, the researchers were able to classify the contractures as being either static or dynamic in nature. If the limitation in movement remained the contracture was said to be static. If the contracture disappeared it was considered to be dynamic.

When the muscles were biopsied the gastrocnemius and biceps femoris muscles showed the least changes. One could assume (ignoring individual differences) that these muscles are predominately composed of type _____ muscle fibers.

II

---

130. Dynamic contractures were found in the vastus medialis; that is under anesthesia the vastus medialis muscles could be taken through the joint range of motion. Muscle biopsies showed atrophy of both type I and type II muscle fibers.

It might be expected that biopsy results would be different in muscles with dynamic contractures as compared to muscles with _____ contractures.

static

131. Static contractures were noted in muscles which are usually said to be predominately type I, that is, the soleus and the anterior and posterior tibalis muscles, had some static contractures.

In these muscles, type I **atrophy** was noted along with hypertrophy of type _____ fibers.

II

---

132. The adductor muscles, on the other hand, showed definite static contractures and type I muscle fiber hypertrophy.

Such studies tell us that it is difficult to generalize findings from individual to individual with spasticity, but also from muscle to muscle, even in the presence of fiber type predominance.

Thus, it would seem logical that all types of "spastic muscles" may not respond to the same _____.

treatment

---

133. Perhaps the most important observation to make from this information is that the presence of spasticity produces profound alterations in muscle.

The muscle is also most likely to be the most change-able (mutable) tissue relative to our _____ programs.

treatment

---

134. Early treatment intervention, however, may prevent or minimize the influences responsible for producing the undesirable alterations in nervous system function as well as changes in the _____ fibers.

muscle

135. A study by Tardieu, et.al. in 1982 involved children with cerebral palsey who had spastic hypoextensibility of the triceps surae muscles. Hypoextensibility was defined as increased resistance in noncontracting muscle. The children could be divided into two different groups relative to the pathomechanisms causing the hypoextensibility.

In one group of children the shortness of the muscles was attributed to primary defective trophic regulation. In such cases the growth of the muscle did not keep up with the growth of the bone.

Ultimately, the bone will become _____ than the muscle.

longer

---

136. Children who have hypoextensibility of the triceps surae muscles caused by defective trophic regulation responded well to surgical elongation of the tendon. These children failed to respond to muscle lengthening treatment such as casting.

This study by Tardieu, et.al. (1982) illustrates the necessity for classifying patients. If the apparent symptoms or findings result from different pathomechanisms, it is likely the patients will respond to different types of _____.

treatment

---

137. The Tardieu study showed that children with cerebral palsey who had hypoextensibility of the triceps surae muscles because of a primary defective trophic regulation responded best to _____ treatment.

surgical

138. In a second group of children the muscle hypoexten-sibility was related to primary imbalance between the action of the triceps surae and dorsiflexor muscles. Prolonged activity of the plantar flexor muscles produces shortening of the that group.

Children with this muscle imbalance responded well to muscle lengthening by successive plaster casting.

As might be expected, this group did not respond well to _____ treatment.

surgical

---

139. It is clear from this research that all cases of hypoextensibility of the plantar flexor muscles cannot be effectively treated in the same manner. These children may appear to have the same problem, but the outward signs do not reflect a common neuropathology.

If the underlying mechanisms of the disorder are not the same, it should not be surprising that treatment results from one child cannot be _____ to another.

generalized

---

140. For years researchers and clinicians alike have searched for methods to quantify muscle "tone." This term is no longer significant and may be irrelevant and misleading.

Because the state of resistance in a spastic muscle varies with any number of influences (position, emotions, resistance, etc.) the manual muscle test surely has no validity or reliability.

Some experimental protocols have provided data that may prove useful in further attempts to "measure" _____.

spasticity

141. Burke, et.al. (1971) measured the amplitude of EMG response to stretch applied at various velocities.

When the quadriceps muscle is slowly stretched by knee flexion, no EMG response was noted. As the stretch was applied more rapidly the reflex response increased as the velocity increased.

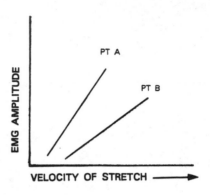

The slope of the EMG and velocity measures could be a relatively objective measure of muscle response. If the electrode placement was standardized, this slope may be a measure of one component of _____ (Bishop, 1977).

spasticity

---

142. This experiment showed that the reflex response must be in the dynamic phase of stretch because no EMG was recorded when the muscle was stretched _____.

slowly

---

143. EMG activity ceases to be recorded when the movement ceases. Therefore, the enhanced reflex response is probably not a result of the _____ phase of stretch.

static

144. Burke, et.al. (1971) also noted that the initial length of the muscle before applying stretch directly affected the amplitude of the EMG. These investigators also noted that flexor muscles responded differently than extensor muscles.

The shorter the initial length of the quadriceps the greater the response to stretch. Conversely, the longer the initial length the greater the response in the _____ muscles.

hamstring

---

145. Burke postulated that this observed response was mediated by the secondary ending. Whether this supposition is true or false, the results point out once again some differences between some _____ and _____ muscles.

flexor
extensor

---

146. Many questions have arisen relative to the effectiveness of stretch in the treatment of spasticity. We have long known that rapid or abrupt stretch will most likely produce adverse effects.

Clinicians have also long observed that slow and maintained stretch may have beneficial results. We have already noted that prolonged stretch such as casting is effective with patients with particular types of neuropathology which underlies their motor abnormalities (Tardieu, et.al., 1982).

It is apparent once again that the ability to describe patient problems accurately and to then categorize the pathophysiologic causes of their disorders will determine the effectiveness of _____ selection.

treatment

147. A study was done in which spastic paraplegic patients were placed on a tilt table with the ankle in dorsiflexion. The body weight thus provided a maintained stretch on the plantar flexors (Odeen and Knutsson, 1981).

Standing in this position for 30 minutes produced a marked reduction in the resistance to dorsiflexion. These effects were sustained for a variable period depending on the individual; some for as long as four hours.

Patients were also placed in plantar flexion and some were braced in dorsiflexion and placed supine. The change in resistance in these situations was not significant.

Possibly weight-bearing positions provide a most effective mode of applying _____.

stretch

---

148. Experimental results and empirical observations tell us that appropriately applied stretch can temporarily reduce the effects of _____.

spasticity

---

149. The question is what are the **appropriate** modes of stretch.

Casting, weight-bearing postures and manual stretching are but some possibilities. Whether these will be effective, once again, depends upon a number of variables such as method of applying any mode of stretch and the particular patient to whom the stretch is applied, and perhaps to the particular muscles involved.

Weight-bearing stretch to the plantar flexors has been shown to be effective in some _____ patients.

paraplegic

SUMMARY

A long held view that spasticity is the result of a release phenomenon has been based on acute animal experiments and does not bear a true resemblance to the slow development of spasticity in man.

The classical experiments seemed to indicate that the lack of suppression from descending tracts resulted in either excessive input to alpha neurons or gamma neurons. Thus, one would expect that spasticity could result from excessive fusimotor drive. This drive would produce an increased output from the spindle afferents which, in turn, results in excessive drive on the alpha motor neurons.

While the possibility of excessive fusimotor drive in spasticity has not been irrefutably disproved, research strongly indicates that such excessive drive is not present in disorders of muscle contractibility. It must be remembered that the stretch reflex is not strong enough to drive alpha motor neurons.

Stretch reflexes are present and can be manipulated. The clinician does not imagine that stretch to a spastic muscle augments the response. It most certainly does. The mechanism by which these reflexes are magnified are most likely through changes in the gain or level of sensitivity of the interneuron pool.

The muscle spindle itself is not hyperactive. When a spastic muscle is stretched the extra input from the spindle is added to the already heightened excitability of the central circuits. The spindle itself is not more sensitive in this state. In the past, we have based therapeutic intervention on the premise of being able to "bias" the muscle spindle to new lengths. If its sensitivity has not changed, then "biasing" cannot be done.

One of the problems that may occur in patients with spasticity is the inability to rapidly generate muscle contractions and to "shut off" the contraction at the appropriate time. Continued contractions are most likely maintained by reverberations within the interneuron circuits.

Patients who manifest spasticity do not all behave in the same manner. Some approaches used to reduce spasticity are casting, surgery, drugs, weight-bearing and other forms of maintained stretch. Positions or devices which alleviate rapid and abrupt stretches, lowering the skin temperature and exercising in rotational patterns have also been shown to diminish spasticity. Whether these approaches will be successful depends upon the manner in which they are applied and the individual upon whom they are tried. The ability to classify patients into categories which reflect similar neuropathological mechanisms, responses and so forth should increase our success rate as treatment becomes more appropriate for each individual.

150. It has been well documented that muscle spindle primary (Ia) receptors are very sensitive to vibration. As the vibrator oscillates a small stretch is applied to the muscle and thus to the receptors (Mountcastle, 1980).

Three events occur as a result of this vibration (Bishop 1982; Burke 1983).

One, impulses through the monosynaptic reflex arc facilitate the alpha motor neurons of the agonist and its synergists. If the excitation is sufficient and asynchronous, a slowly building contraction occurs. The contraction is maintained as long as the stimlulus is _____.

maintained

---

151. Two, motor neurons to the antagonists are inhibited. This would be expected through the mechanism of _____ inhibition.

reciprocal

---

152. Three, phasic stretch reflexes are inhibited in the muscle which is vibrated.

A phasic reflex which should be supressed during vibration would be a _____ _____.

tendon tap

---

153. Three events which occur in response to maintained vibration are:
1. _____
2. _____
3. _____

contraction is maintained
antagonists are inhibited
phasic stretch reflexes are inhibited

248

154. The tonic vibration reflex (TVR) is not simply another mechanism for eliciting a stretch reflex. Unlike the stretch reflex the TVR requires additional support from higher centers, as well as multisynaptic spinal mechanisms.

The TVR is not simply a _____-synaptic reflex.

mono

---

155. Normal individuals can voluntarily enhance or suppress the tonic vibration reflex. Since it appears that neither of these events is associated with a change in spindle discharge there must be some central gain-controlling mechanism independent of the muscle _____.

spindle

---

156. In spastic patients the tonic vibration reflex begins abruptly rather than becoming slowly augmented. The spastic patient cannot enhance or suppress the reflex voluntarily as can the normal individual.

This finding further suggests that there is a disturbance of central gain-controlling mechanisms in spasticity which appear to be independent of the _____ system.

fusimotor

---

157. Because the patient with motor disturbances may lack the ability to voluntarily supress the tonic vibration reflex, the extent of voluntary supression may provide a quantitative assessment of motor dysfunction (Bishop, 1982).

In spastic patients, the onset of the tonic vibration reflex is _____.

abrupt

249

158. Some cautions must be made relative to the TVR. Variability in reflex response has been noted in normal man. A TVR may be demonstrable in only some muscles. A TVR does not develop in all normal subjects if they are relaxed.

If there is variability among normal subjects, one might expect variability among _____.

patients

---

159. It may be possible to utilize the TVR response as an evaluation tool.

Patients with motor disturbances may not be able to voluntarily suppress the tonic vibration reflex.

A quantitative measure of motor dysfunction may be extrapolated from the extent of _____ _____ of the TVR.

voluntary suppression

---

160. In spite of the variability of responses, vibration is often a very useful tool in patient treatment and possibly in patient evaluation.

A vibrator may be used to activate muscle which is a proprioceptive response; or to drive pacinian corpuscles in the skin and subcutaneous tissues as an exteroceptive stimulus.

The method of vibrator application will determine its clinical success and effectiveness.

Vibration which is intended to be a **proprioceptive** stimulus (as opposed to exteroceptive) may be applied directly to the muscle belly. Some clinicians prefer to vibrate the tendon or the myotendonous junction. Most importantly, the point of the vibrator should be positioned gently but firmly and held in place. Remember it takes time for the TVR to _____ up.

build

161. Moving a vibrator rapidly up and down a muscle or loosely on the skin will not likely elicit a _____ _____ _____.

tonic vibration
reflex

---

162. Remember that not all normal individuals exhibit tonic vibration reflexes so your patient may not either. One method that will enhance the probability of getting or augmenting a response is to place the muscle to be vibrated in a position of stretch.

With this positioning we may assure that the small stretches will be picked up more likely by the muscle receptors. Excessive length, however, may inhibit the TVR. Each muscle may have an optimum length.

The antagonists to the vibrated muscle will usually be _____.

inhibited

---

163. Excessive length of the muscle which is being vibrated may _____ the TVR.

inhibit

---

164. Vibration responses can also be enhanced by active muscle contraction (Hagbarth & Eklund, 1966; 1968). Increasing levels of voluntary contraction increase the TVR accordingly. Isometric contractions tend to be more effective than isotonic contractions, particularly in somewhat lengthened ranges.

Experiment with each patient and with each muscle to determine the optimum conditions to elicit the desired _____.

response

165. Each muscle may have an optimum length at which the best response occurs when the muscle is _____.

vibrated

---

166. The state or mood of the individual can enhance or depress the TVR (Hagbarth & Eklund, 1968). The level of excitability and cooperation will thus also affect the effectiveness of vibration.

Do not expect all patients with nervous system pathology to react in the same manner. Not only are there individual differences, but patients with different disorders (Parkinson's disease vs. spinal cord injury, for example) will produce _____ reactions.

different

---

167. The choice of vibrators is also important. Effective vibration is usually about 100 to 200 cycles per second (H_2). A significant displacement of the vibrating head is also important. An amplitude of 1.0 to 2.5 mm is the most effective (Homma, et.al., 1967; Johnson, et.al., 1970).

Small battery driven "personal" vibrators often do not have sufficient power or excursion to provide effective vibration. This is particularly true when the vibrator is applied to adults.

Battery vibrators may provide adequate vibration if the patient is a _____.

child

---

168. If the batteries are not fresh the rate of vibration will decrease. Too low a frequency may inhibit the TVR. Frequency will also drop when the vibrator tip is firmly pushed into the _____ belly.

muscle

252

169. The more distal muscles have less tissue bulk over the bony structure. Thus vibration may be picked up through the skeleton and transferred to the antagonistic muscle. This may produce unwanted muscle _____.

contraction

---

170. Electric vibrators exist which may provide sufficient vibratory input. The greatest difficulty is finding one that allows a relatively small point of application. Broad flat vibrator heads are not likely to produce useful proprioceptive stimuli.

To assure appropriate vibratory stimuli, the vibrator head should be _____.

small

---

171. The best way to enhance muscle activity with a vibrator is to apply the vibration **while the muscle is contracting.**

The vibrator must be held firmly for at least 10-15 seconds in one _____.

place

---

172. For effective results, the muscles to be vibrated should be placed in a position of _____.

stretch

173. Additionally, the best responses usually occur if the muscle is _____.

contracting

---

174. Spiral-diagonal movements may enhance the response to vibration (Marsden, et.al., 1969) so, rotational patterns such as those utilized in PNF (proprioceptive neuromuscular facilitation) should be used with vibration.

An excellent way to sustain muscle contraction is to add resistance to the muscle in a diagonal pattern while it is being _____.

vibrated

---

175. Applying ice to the skin to produce mild cooling of the area will also enhance the vibratory response. An unpublished investigation by the authors showed this observation to be true in every case involving normal individuals.

The optimum level of skin cooling may vary with the _____.

individual

---

176. Adverse effects from vibration, in addition to those noted, have also been observed. Patients with motor abnormalities may exhibit increased tremor, rigidity, incoordination and clonus (Hagbarth & Eklund, 1968).

Patients with such diagnoses as hemiplegia, cerebral palsy, spinal cord injury, Parkinson's disease and cerebellar disease may demonstrate different responses to vibration.

Therapists will have to evaluate the responses of each patient to determine the treatment _____.

effectiveness

177. Vibratory responses can be influenced by:

a. _____

b. _____

c. _____

d. _____

e. _____

f. _____

g. _____

h. _____

i. _____

a. muscle length
b. voluntary contraction
c. isometric vs. isotonic contractions
d. state or mood
e. type of pathology
f. individual variability
g. method of vibrator application
h. temperature of the skin
i. bony vs. fleshy areas vibrated

SUMMARY

The primary receptors of the muscle spindle are very sensitive to vibration.

As the vibrator oscillates a small stretch is applied to the muscle and thus to the receptors. If the excitation is sufficient, a slowly building contraction occurs which is maintained as long as the vibration is maintained. This response is referred to as the tonic vibration reflex (TVR).

The TVR utilizes the stretch reflex but also requires additional support from higher centers.

In spastic patients the TVR usually begins abruptly rather than as a slowly augmenting response. The spastic patient cannot voluntarily enhance or suppress the TVR as can the normal individual. The amount of voluntary suppression may be useful as a quantitative assessment in patients with motor abnormalities.

Tonic vibration can be a very useful tool in patient treatment and evaluation. An effective vibrator must be chosen and the vibrator must be applied appropriately to elicit the desired response.

For muscle activation, the vibrator should be pressed firmly but not too deeply on the muscle (or tendon) and held in place to allow the contraction to build. The response may be enhanced if the muscle is contracting or placed on a stretch.

There are numerous conditions or situations which will influence the result of vibration. Some of these are:

a. muscle length
b. voluntary contraction
c. isometric vs. isotonic contractions
d. state or mood
e. type of pathology
f. individual variability
g. method of vibrator application
h. temperature of the skin
i. bony vs. fleshy areas vibrated

As conditions and patients vary, it is necessary to experiment with every patient and observe the patient's response to determine whether vibration will be effective in each case.

CO-CONTRACTION

178. The concept we will now investigate is that of co-contraction or co-activation of agonists and antagonists. There has been much discussion surrounding the application and definition of what therapists call "co-contraction."

Basmajian (1978) defines co-contraction as "the simultaneous contraction of both the agonists (or prime movers) and the antagonists, with a supremacy of the former producing the visible motion." This means that while the joint is visibly performing extension, both extensors and _____ may be contracting.

flexors

---

179. Both the flexor and the extensor muscles may contract simultaneously in _____.

co-contraction

---

180. The achievement of co-contraction does not necessarily imply that a joint must be in a static position as was once thought. Although both the agonist and antagonist are contracting simultane-ously, visible motion may occur. This is due to the supremacy of the _____ of the movement.

agonists

---

181. Co-contraction is the co-activation of _____ and _____.

agonists
antagonists

182. For hundreds of years it was believed that the antagonist must **always** be completely relaxed (reciprocal innervation) for the agonist or prime mover to contract. Galen, the great physiologist of antiquity maintained this view, and was not refuted until Duchenne wrote of quite different observations in 1866.

Duchenne argued that human joints and motions were too complex for reciprocal activity to produce coordinated movement. He maintained that "moderating and collateral muscular associations" or "harmony of the antagonists" was necessary to provide adequate control (Duchenne, 1949).

It is interesting that controversy over this topic should continue to modern times.

"Harmony of the antagonists" is a definition of _____ in Duchenne's terms.

co-contraction

---

183. There are many conflicting studies and opinions about co-contraction. One indicates that co-contraction occurs only in resisted movement, and another suggests that co-contraction occurs during unresisted movement.

Some writers say that it occurs in skilled activity; others favor gross activities, and still others argue that co-contraction occurs only during stabilizing postural functions.

Patton and Mortenson (1971) investigated co-contraction, using electromyographic recordings, in an attempt to clarify these conflicting reports.

Duchenne defined co-contraction as "harmony of the _____."

antagonists

---

184. Many conclusions about co-contraction have been made using assumptions based on observations and some known, but perhaps irrelevant physiological facts.

EMG studies were done to provide more direct information concerning _____.

co-contraction

185. Patton noted that simultaneous contraction of muscles on both sides of the joint could occur during voluntary movement.

The interplay of primary (Ia), secondary (II), and GTO (Ib) nerve fiber responses possibly provides some basis for co-contraction.

Co-contraction is simultaneous contraction of agonists and antagonists with supremacy of the agonists producing the _____ motion.

desired

---

186. Patton's study noted that the incidence and degree of co-contraction was greater during extension movements than _____ movements.

flexion

---

187. Physical and occupational therapists believed there was value in promoting co-contraction in patients with apparent deficits in stability. Equally important has been the need to discover or define the physiological basis of this activity. Co-contraction can be achieved by higher center controls. In this text we will explore only the contributions from the peripheral system.

In the past, the peripheral basis for co-contraction had been assigned to the secondary (II) ending because they were thought to be excitatory only to flexor muscles and inhibitory to extensors.

Thus, if this were true, a stretch of the extensor muscles should produce _____.

co-contraction

259

188. As some secondary (II) fibers supplying muscle afferents do contribute to the flexor reflexes and in general produce inhibition in extensor groups, it is possible that secondary receptors of the muscle spindle do, therefore, contribute to _____.

co-contraction

189. Because many secondary receptors make monosynaptic excitatory synapses on their own muscles whether they are flexors or extensors, these receptors are unlikely to provide the total explanation for the phenomenon of _____.

co-contraction

190. Therapists of almost any level of clinical experience have clearly seen the activation of flexor muscles when stretching extensor muscles. One very effective procedure is to have the patient squat to put a full stretch on the soleus. Then the patient is urged to attempt to return to standing. If the range through which the patient is permitted to move is restricted, activation of the dorsiflexors can be seen.

Quite possibly some of this response is explained by the elicitation of equilibrium reactions in the feet (see **The Neurophysiological Basis of Patient Treatment, Vol. II Reflexes in Motor Development** by Barnes, Crutchfield, and Heriza).

It is also possible that some contribution to this clinical observation is likely to come from the multisynaptic group of secondary (II) receptors that are located in the _____ muscles.

extensor

191. Some secondary receptors may make multisynaptic connections which are specifically inhibitory to _____.

extensors

192. The GTO may contribute most significantly to the phenomenon of co-contraction. First, you will recall that the GTO (Ib) afferent effects are far more widespread in extensors than in flexors (Kandel, 1981).

Therefore, if an extensor is strongly **activated** the result could be _____ of the extensors and _____ of the flexors.

inhibition
facilitation

---

193. Recall also that the GTO will produce strong inhibition when its own muscle is undergoing **active** contraction while the muscle is in a relatively lengthened position.

These conditions are met when, for instance, the soleus muscle is fully lengthened and contracting during a deep _____.

squat

---

194. During this squat the soleus (extensor) is stretched while actively contracting and is inhibited. By reciprocal innervation the tibilalis anterior muscle is _____.

excited

---

195. It has been observed by many therapists of the authors' acquaintance, that co-contraction patterns are stimulated best when the patient is weight-bearing. This activity "fixes" the point of insertion of the muscle much more than when the distal part of the extremity is non-weight bearing and "free".

Quite possibly, such a treatment pattern will have a greater infuence on activation of _____ receptors.

GTO (Ib)

196. GTO receptors (Ib) have been found to be very active when the distal attachment is "fixed" and the muscle is in a lengthened position while undergoing active _____.

contraction

---

197. Most likely this enhancement of GTO function under these conditions explains why it is often best elicited under weight bearing conditions rather than non-weightbearing with the distal attachments of the extremity "free" or with passive _____.

stretch

---

198. Co-contraction is best elicited by stretching or contracting the _____ muscles.

extensor

---

199. It has been suggested that joint compression will facilitate co-contraction. Such a response would most likely be mediated by joint receptors.

As a weight-bearing position would compress the associated joints, this mechanism may also contribute to _____.

co-contraction

---

200. Co-contraction may be best elicited by utilizing a _____ position.

weight-bearing

201. It has been observed that, in the early stages of learning a new skill, much co-contraction is present around a joint, and this activity decreases with greater proficiency with the skill (O'Connell and Gardner, 1967).

For the purposes of patient treatment and evaluation, co-contraction may be defined as a balance of muscular tone around the joint which will provide a stable base permitting movement to occur in any direction. Activation of the GTO (Ib) receptors in an extensor muscle may produce _____.

co-contraction

---

202. Co-contraction appears in the early stages of _____ _____.

learning a new skill

---

203. It has long been believed that stability at a joint (particularly proximal joints) is necessary before distal **skilled** activity is possible. Such joint stability may be achieved by _____ (Stockmeyer, 1967).

co-contraction

---

204. With flexor activation a great portion of the facilitation is on one side of the joint. This produces further activation of flexors (and inhibition of extensors).

In this situation it is likely that there is little possibility for _____.

co-contraction

263

205. The Patton study also noted that co-contraction increased with increasing loads, and no evidence was presented to indicate that it increased with more precise movements. Actually, less co-contraction was recorded when the more skilled or strong individuals were tested.

Thus co-contraction is probably a more "primitive" activity than skill, and may be necessary as a basis for early developmental patterns for _____.

skill

_____

206. If the extensor muscles can be activated, it may be possible to facilitate the _____ muscles through them.

flexors

_____

207. Co-contraction may occur if the stretch and GTO reflexes are activated in _____ muscles.

extensor

_____

208. Such co-contraction activity may be initiated even in the presence of little function. This activity is present through all levels of achievements including those of normal individuals.

If flexor activity is already powerful, the extensor muscle should be activated **first** to prevent inhibition from active flexors. This will condition the extensors to generate tension. Such an approach is a particular necessity when treatment involves spastic upper extremities.

Through reciprocal innervation if the flexors are activated, the _____ will be inhibited.

extensors

209. When treating patients with spasticity in the lower extremities you may wish to improve the tension generated by the extensors first or you may go directly to squat-stance activities if the extensors are sufficiently _____.

strong or active

---

210. If the extensors are activated first, the flexors may be enhanced by placing a stretch on the extensors while they are contracting in order to fire the _____ and _____ receptors.

secondary and GTO

---

211. In patient treatment, it is useful to activate the extensors before permitting flexor activity. Once the extensor can produce maintained activity, it can be stretched under tension and will activate its own GTO (Ib) and possibly secondary receptors which will facilitate the flexor. Therefore, imbalance in muscle strength may be eliminated or modified when _____ is produced at the joint.

co-contraction

---

212. With advanced practice and acquisition of skill less and less co-contraction may be required.

Co-contraction may be important and a particular goal in patient treatment because without stability at proximal joints there may be difficulty in achieving some _____ movements.

skilled

213. As therapists, we may have been overly concerned with co-contraction or may have misinterpreted the findings presented by our patients. The patients' inability to produce a distal movement may not be solely, or even partially, because of a lack of co-contraction at proximal joints.

Suppose the patient is on a tilt board. When he is tilted one way the knee buckles. Tilted the other way the knee hyperextends and the patient falls off the board. The assumptions made by the therapist are that something is wrong with the vestibular reflex and that the patient has a problem with co-contraction of the trunk as he lacks proximal stability.

So the treatment is not based on the therapist's observations, but rather on the therapist's assumptions (Horak, 1984).

Patients may appear to have "proximal instability" and yet have no problem from the standpoint of producing _____.

co-contraction

----

214. Much of coordinated movement consists of pre-programmed patterns which do not require sensory input or feedback to be activated. Movement has a part which is voluntary and a part which is reflex (Horak, 1984).

When a normal individual lifts an arm rapidly in a straight arm raise, EMG recordings show that the first muscle activity is in the paraspinals and biceps femoris muscles on the contralateral side.

EMG studies on stroke patients show that their inability to raise the uninvolved arm is the result of the inability to generate enough tension in these preparatory muscles on the involved side (Horak, 1984).

Excessive background noise or tension was not noted as we have come to believe would happen if the patient had _____.

spasticity

215. In the case of the forward arm lift, the lack of proximal stability occurred because of the decrease in preparatory muscle activity.

The patient, who may be spastic, cannot raise his arm because of the inability to generate adequate muscle tension in the _____ muscles.

paraspinal

---

216. Timing of muscle activity also contributes to coordinated movement. A response may require the orderly and sequential activation of certain muscles. For instance, to maintain posture the gastrocnemius may be activated followed by the hamstring and the paraspinals.

In this case the stabilizing muscles are not the proximal muscles, but rather the _____ muscles.

distal

---

217. If the muscles are not activated in the appropriate sequence the individual demonstrates postural movement abnormalities.

This sequence of activity may begin in the _____ muscles.

distal

---

218. Co-contraction or co-activation may not be present when the individual is the most stable. We have already noted that co-contraction decreases with the acquisition of _____.

skill

267

219. It is important as therapists to learn that patients must be carefully observed during treatment and that results in one patient cannot be generalized to other patients.

As we learn more about the components of normal coordinated movement, treatment rationales must be altered.

All movements do not begin with _____ stability.

proximal

---

220. Our job as therapists in such situations will be to help the patient gain a normal movement _____.

sequence

---

221. One must not discard the concept that without proximal stability, distal mobility is difficult, altered or impossible. If a hip muscle is weak the individual will have difficulty standing or walking. The major point is that "stability" does not usually mean "co-contraction."

Emphasis on proximal muscles in treatment certainly has its place. If the distal muscle begins the movement and the proximal muscles follow there will be obvious abnormalities if the latter are weak.

Good treatment programs require careful observation and the ability of the therapist to change treatment based on those observations. It is very easy to assume that proximal muscles are weak or co-contraction is lacking by observing certain behaviors.

Treatment programs begin to fail when they are not based on observations, but rather on _____.

assumptions

SUMMARY

Co-contraction or co-activation has been defined as "the simultaneous contraction of both the agonists and antagonists, with a supremacy of the former producing the visible motor" (Basmajian, 1978).

Patton and Mortenson (1971) observed that co-contraction could occur during voluntary movement. The incidence and degree of co-contraction is greater during extension movements. Co-contraction has also been observed during the initial stages of learning a new skill. As the skill becomes refined, co-contraction decreases or ceases to be observed.

In the past the physiological basis for co-contraction has been assigned to the secondary receptor of the muscle spindle because it was believed to be exclusively excitatory to flexor muscles and inhibitory to extensor muscles. Thus, activating an extensor would result in excitation of the extensor muscles (primary ending) and also the flexor muscles (secondary ending).

It has been shown that the secondary ending is not exclusively excitatory to flexor muscles. There are some A beta-gamma (II) size fibers which are found in nerves to the muscles which do facilitate flexors and these fibers may or may not come from the muscle spindle.

The GTO may assist in mediating co-contraction. Its effects are far more widespread in extensor muscles than flexor muscles. Thus, strong activation of extensors would produce strong inhibition of extensors and excitation of flexors. As contraction of a relatively elongated and "fixed" muscle results in vigorous firing of the GTO, weight-bearing activities such as deep squats may produce the strongest co-contraction patterns.

As therapists we must be cautious in applying exercise patterns designed to elicit co-contraction and develop proximal stability. Co-activation may not be present in the most stable patterns and may, in fact, be present in unstable conditions. Additionally, the appropriate pattern of muscle activation in a desired activity may begin distally. The stability for the movement would, therefore, be distal rather than proximal in these cases. Undoubtedly, the condition of proximal muscles will remain a concern as for many movements the proximal muscle fix and stabilize the proximal joints to allow distal movement to take place.

222. Have you wondered why most terminology concerning muscles relates to "flexors" and "extensors"? What happened to adductors and rotators? In some cases, of course, such actions are combined by muscles acting over a multiaxial joint. For example, the pectoralis major is a shoulder flexor--and also an adductor and internal rotator by virtue of its attachment across a multiaxial joint.

Muscles are often classified into two groups. So far we can say that one of these groups contains flexors and the other contains _____.

extensors

---

223. Embryologically, muscles arise from myotomes which correspond to the spinal root levels. As development continues, some myotomes fuse with others and some degenerate. This is how a muscle becomes innervated by more than one _____ segment.

spinal

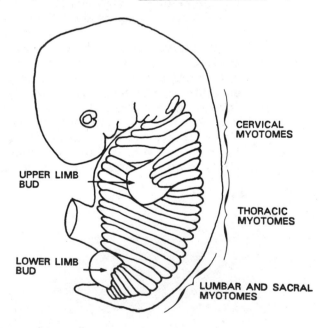

224. As the myotomes develop into muscles they become arranged in one of two ways. Those placed ventrally and pre-axially (in front of the skeleton) become flexors and will be innervated by anterior divisions of the plexuses innervating them. **Adductors** and **internal rotators** also are formed by the same masses and are innervated in the same manner. Group 1 muscles, then, are flexors, _____, and _____ _____ (Patton, 1953).

adductors
internal rotators

VERTEBRA

BACK MUSCLES

APPENDICULAR SKELETON

POST-AXIAL MUSCLES (EXTENSORS, ETC.)

CHEST WALL MUSCLES

PRE-AXIAL MUSCLES (FLEXORS, ETC.)

225. The myotomes located posteriorly and post-axially become **extensors** and are innervated by posterior divisions of their plexuses. **Abductors and external rotators** are also formed and innervated accordingly (Patten, 1953).

Group 2 muscles consist of extensors, _____, and _____ _____.

abductors
external rotators

226. Rotation of the limb buds in human embryos has complicated the picture. However, a closer look at the innervations will show flexors, adductors, and internal rotators (Group _____ muscles) to be generally innervated by the same segments. The same is true for Group _____ muscles.

1
2

271

227. You will also recall that physiologists simply named all anti-gravity muscles as extensors. Anti-gravity muscles may also include abductors and _____ _____.

external
rotators

---

228. Group 2 muscles are _____
_____
_____

extensors
abductors
external rotators

---

229. It appears logical then, that if a flexor is specifically influenced by a certain innervation others in the group will behave in the same manner. If the secondary endings are facilitatory to flexors they also facilitate _____, _____
_____ muscles.

adductors
internal rotator

---

230. Group 1 muscles are the antagonists to Group 2. Therefore, Group 1, if activated may inhibit Group 2 by _____ _____.

reciprocal
innervation

---

231. "Physiological" flexors are antagonists of anti-_____ muscles.

gravity

232. Anti-gravity muscles are often referred to as "physiological" _____.

extensors

---

233. If muscles are grouped as physiological flexors and extensors they may not necessarily fall in the same category as they would with our Group I and Group II classifications.

A muscle in the upper extremity would be classified differently than one in the _____ _____.

lower extremity

---

234. Two joint muscles are more difficult to classify.

A two joint muscle may flex at one joint and extend at another and in that sense could be both a Group 1 and a Group 2 muscle. Two joint muscles that flex at both joints or extend at both joints apparently fall within their respective categories.

Because it extends at both the shoulder and elbow joints, the triceps brachii is probably a Group _____ muscle.

2

---

235. Two joint muscles present multiple problems because they have actions over more than one joint and are generally classified as more phasic in nature. A two joint muscle may be a flexor at one joint and an extensor at another and, therefore, classified as both a Group _____ and Group _____ muscle.

1
2

273

236. A better term for a two joint extensor which will be coined at this time is a two joint **hybrid*** muscle. Technically, if the muscle flexes at one joint and exends at the other, it cannot be classified totally as a two joint flexor or a two joint extensor. It also cannot be exclusively classified as a physiological flexor or extensor.

In this volume two joint muscles with opposing functions at each joint will be termed two joint _____ muscles.

hybrid

*American Heritage Dictionary definition of hybrid— Something of mixed origin or composition.

---

237. Although it may have no anatomical or physiological relevance, from a functional standpoint we can refer to muscles as falling in one of 3 catgories: Group _____, Group _____ and _____ _____ _____.

1
2
two joint hybrids

---

238. Clinical therapists have tried for years to implicate Group 1 muscles as those most likely to become involved with nervous system disorders. They believed that spasticity would be most prevalent in flexors, adductors and internal rotators.

Because some of the two joint hybrid muscles are usually also involved, therapists also attempted to place them in Group _____.

1

239. Individuals familiar with gait problems, particularly in spastic disorders, are fully aware of the difficulty in treatment when a spastic or shortened gastrocnemius muscle is encountered.

Through a reflex system, any pressure on the ball of the foot results in an exaggerated positive supporting reaction. This probably involves participation of **all** plantar flexors, however, as the gastrocnemius also crosses the knee joint other complications arise.

All plantar flexors may be involved in the extensor thrust reflex or exaggerated positive supporting reaction, however, only the _____ crosses two joints.

gastrocnemius

---

240. Two joint muscles are more superficial and tend to be more phasic in nature than one joint muscles. Therefore, the activation of these muscles would be less likely to produce the **maintained** or **tonic** activity desired in patient treatment than would one joint muscles (O'Connell and Gardner, 1972).

An example of a two joint phasic muscle is the _____.

gastrocnemius

---

241. Individuals in clinical practice have attempted to "drive" the dorsiflexors of the ankle by placing a maintained stretch on the plantar flexors (extensors) to achieve co-contraction at the ankle.

This often works well if the knee is flexed and no pressure is allowed on the ball of the foot, but an exaggerated positive supporting reflex occurs immediately if done with the knee extended. Thus, the conclusion has often been that as the gastrocnemius cannot be used to activate dorsiflexors it must not be a Group 2 muscle.

It has been classified, therefore, as a Group 1 muscle because it "behaves as a _____."

flexor

242. Clinical problems may arise primarily with two joint hybrid muscles (these are generally the gastrocnemius, rectus femoris and hamstring muscles). Of these, the gastrocnemius is probably the greatest offender.

Actually, the authors believe that the positive supporting reflex can be elicited when the leg is in position to stretch the gastrocnemius muscle (dorsiflexion with knee extension) simply because this position tends to enhance the entire extensor synergy pattern which predominates in the lower extremity.

Flexing the knee helps to prevent this by releasing some stretch on the gastrocneumius muscle, and therefore, one link in the synergy pattern is removed.

The gastrocnemius adds particular problems to the extensor synergy pattern because it crosses the _____ joint.

knee

---

243. The complication of treatment by activation of the gastrocnemius muscle is probably rests with the following facts: (1) it involves more than one joint (which always complicates movement), (2) it is primarily a phasic muscle and, therefore, not easily utilized for tonic activation and (3) the position necessary for its activation tends to facilitate the entire extensor synergy in the lower extremity.

It is **not** valid to classify the gastrocnemius (and other two joint extensors) as a Group I muscle **on the premise** that it "behaves as a _____."

flexor

244. As we have noted, a careful look at the distribution of spasticity in just about any neurologically involved patient will show that Group 1 distribution of spasticity does not hold up under scrutiny.

Group 1 muscles in the upper extremity are likely to be spastic, however, Group 2 muscles are usually involved in the _____ extremity.

lower

---

245. Spasticity is actually more pronounced in muscles we have already described as "physiological extensors". These are muscles which are _____ muscles.

anti-gravity

---

246. Anti-gravity muscles of the upper extremity are _____.

flexors

---

247. Anti-gravity muscles of the lower extremity are _____.

extensors

---

248. An important reason for you to be aware of these discrepancies is that authors often fail to indicate what they mean by "flexors" and "extensors." It follows that the clinician will have difficulty interpreting such information. If the author and the clinician are referring to opposite muscles as being flexors it is no wonder some clinical results appear to be the exact opposite of the "facts" on which they were based.

Careful observation on the part of the therapist will minimize any adverse effects from misinterpretation of the _____.

literature

277

249. Some information about range of motion may be helpful at this time. We will consider the **maximum** and **submaximum** portions of the full range.

There is a maximum range for both flexor and extensor muscles as well as the other Group 1 and Group 2 muscles.

Each flexor and extensor muscle has a _____ range.

maximum

---

250. The extent of the range of motion in which a flexor is on **maximum stretch** or length is the _____ range of the flexor.

maximum

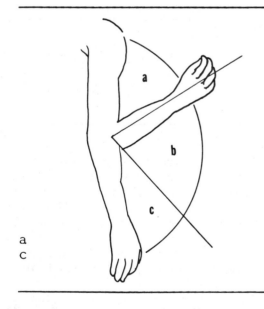

251. Consider the drawing as representing the normal range of motion; the maximum range for the extensor is _____ (a, b, or c).

Maximum range for the flexor is _____ (a, b, or c).

a
c

---

252. In the c range illustrated in the last frame, the flexors are on _____ stretch.

maximum

253. As the movement is reversed and the elbows comes into flexion, there will be a point where the extensors are on maximum stretch.

This is the _____ range of the extensors.

maximum

---

254. The center zone, which usually contains the greatest percentage of the total range of motion, is termed the submaximum range for both flexors and extensors.

The area where neither the flexor nor the extensor is on maximum stretch is called _____ range for both.

submaximum

---

255. The quadriceps are activated the most strongly at a short initial length. The hamstrings are activated most when they are at the longest initial length (Burke, et.al., 1971).

Whether the mechanism for this phenomenon rests with the secondary ending, inhibition of the hamstrings may be more effectively accomplished by activating the quadriceps in the _____ range.

submaximum

---

256. It is not always possible to generalize from the findings just reviewed. Until research is completed on different muscles we cannot say that the biceps and triceps muscles in the upper extremity behave exactly as those muscles studied in the _____ extremity.

lower

257. As was noted previously, the secondary (II) receptor which is active throughout the range fires with greater frequency near the physiological limit of the muscle.

Therefore, it is possible that greater responses may occur in the _____ range.

maximum

---

258. The secondary afferent (II) fibers most likely produce two different effects. The monosynaptic terminals produce excitation of their own muscle.

The monosynoptic secondary afferent (II) fiber contributes to the _____ _____ reflex.

tonic stretch

---

259. There are some nerve fibers of the II class size which make multisynaptic connections with their motor neurons and are most likely associated with flexor reflexes. Activation of flexor reflexes would be inhibitory to extensors.

Both the secondary (II) receptor and the GTO (Ib) would be more active at the extremes of range. If you want maximum extensor excitation, it would be best to exercise them in the _____ range.

sub-maximum

---

260. Thus, if the treatment objective is to increase output from the extensors, it may be prudent to avoid activating them in the _____ range.

maximum

280

261. If the extensors are contracting in the submaximum range, it is less likely that any multisynaptic secondary (II) receptors in the extensor will be strongly activated.

Don't forget that the greatest effects from the GTO occur in contracting _____ muscles.

extensor

262. The GTO's are also strongly activated when the muscle is actively contracting while at its greatest length.

Therefore, activating extensors in the maximum range could produce the greatest _____ effects on the extensors.

inhibitory

263. Although the patient may not have a full normal range of motion at a joint, there is still a maximum range for flexors, one for extensors, and a submaximum range for both.

Don't forget individual differences. In two patients with a 30° range of motion, one may have 5° maximum range for flexors and extensors while the other may have 10°.

Even in cases of reduced range of motion, there will be a maximum range for _____ and extensors and _____ _____ for both.

flexors
submaximum range

264. Some of the secondary receptors may be specifically excitatory to flexors and inhibitory to extensors. These receptors respond with greater intensity in a _____ range.

maximum

281

265. In fact, the exitatory level of the motor neuron pool in question may well determine how rapidly an individual may increase excitation within the range.

Therefore, the **exact** point at which the range becomes maximum may vary from time to time in any individual.

Thus, maximum and submaximum ranges are **not** likely to be _____ entities.

static, set, or
unchanging

---

266. Depending on the central program in operation, this secondary receptor activation in the maximum range may overwhelm the activity of the static _____ _____ fibers.

primary afferent

---

267. Four ways which may favor excitation of the flexor muscles and inhibit the extensors by stretch or repetitive input might be (state which muscle group is to be stretched):

1. quick stretch to flexor anywhere in the range
2. maintained stretch or repetitive input to flexor in the submaximum range
3. maintained stretch or repetitive input to flexor in the maximum range
4. maintained stretch or repetitive input to extensor in the maximum range

268. If we consider that a more functional classification of muscles might be "physiological flexors and extensors," the pattern of activation may depend upon the location of the muscle.

The physiological extensor muscles of the upper extremity are the _____.

flexors

_____

269. Careful observation of the patients' responses to such sensory input as stretch and resistance are necessary.

Complex muscles such as the deltoid may behave differently than less complex muscles such as the brachioradialis.

Research findings on the behavior of two muscles located in a particular extremity cannot always be generalized to different muscles in the same extremity or to those in another _____.

extremity

SUMMARY

The terms "flexor" and extensor" have come to mean general classes of muscles whether they have multiple actions (flexor, adductor, internal rotator) or certain different actions (abductor).

Embryologically, the flexors, adductors and internal rotators develop from ventral or pre-axial myotomes, and the extensors, abductors and external rotators from dorsal or post-axial myotomes.

For some purposes it may be useful to classify these muscles into two groups which will be called Group 1 and Group 2 instead of flexors and extensors. Group 1 will consist of flexors, adductors and internal rotators and Group 2 will be their antagonists. Muscles which cross two joints and have opposing functions at those joints have been labeled by the authors as two-joint hybrid muscles. Rather than imply any functional label, this term was selected only to bring to your attention that these superficial two-joint, phasic muscles often complicate or present treatment problems, particularly with the spastic patient.

Physiologists classify muscles as to **physiological extensors** (anti-gravity musculature) and **physiological flexors.** The physiological extensors in the upper extremity are Group 1 muscles, while in the lower extremity they are Group 2. A two-joint hybrid muscle is not exclusively either a physiological flexor or extensor.

This exercise in classification has been done to: (1) illustrate what muscles are associated with the broad terms "flexor" and "extensor," and how abductors, rotators and so forth relate to these terms; (2) show that different systems may be used. Authors often fail to indicate what they mean by these terms. Anyone who wishes to apply information found in the literature must keep the possiblity of misinterpretation in mind; and (3) bring attention to the general patterns of distribution of spasticity.

We can arbitrarily divide the range of motion available at a joint into three zones. There is a zone in which the flexor muscle is at its greatest length (maximum range); a zone in which it is at its shortest and the antagonist is at its greatest length (maximum range for extensors), and an intermediate zone where neither muscle is elongated (submaximum range).

It is important to recognize that the division line between these zones is arbitrary and changeable given the pathology or excitability state at the time. They may be useful as conceptual guidelines for certain aspects of patient treatment.

The primary afferent endings of the muscle spindle respond to quick (dynamic) or maintained stretch (static) anywhere in the range of motion. The secondary receptors (II) are also responsive throughout the range, but produce their greatest frequency near the physiological limits of the muscle (maximum range).

The multisynaptic A beta-gamma (II) size fibers tend to be predominantly excitatory to flexors. Some of these fibers may come from the secondary endings of the muscle spindle. If this is the case, to maintain maximum excitation of extensor muscles it may be useful to avoid their maximum range.

The GTO produces its greatest effects when contracting a muscle while it is in its fully lengthened position. As these effects are most effective in extensors, they provide another reason that you may wish to avoid the maximum range if you wish maximum contraction of the extensor muscles. On the other hand, if co-activation (co-contraction) of the flexor and extensor muscles is desired, working in the maximum range may be helpful.

Therapists must be careful not to generalize research on two muscles to other pairs of muscles in the same lower extremity, and certainly should not assume the results in the lower extremity will be similar to those in an upper extremity.

SECTION IV

Other Peripheral Receptors

1. Other Sensory Receptors in Muscle

2. Joint Receptors

3. Cutaneous Receptors

OTHER SENSORY RECEPTORS IN MUSCLE

1. Within the supportive tissues of muscle are numerous receptors other than the muscle spindle or the Golgi tendon organ. These additional sensory receptors and fibers also take part in innervating other tissues.

   Excluding the muscle spindle and GTO, the types of sensory receptors found in muscle are also found in other _____ of the body.

tissues

---

2. The additional sensory fibers that are found in muscle nerves occupy a wide range of sizes from I to IV or, depending upon the classification system utilized, fibers may range from A to _____.

C

---

3. Actual endings within the muscle have not been unequivocally found for as many as two-thirds of this fiber population (Stacey, 1969).

   According to Wyke (1979) and others, many fibers terminating in the joints course through the muscle and tendon on the way to the joint.

   We cannot be sure that two-thirds of the fibers found in muscle nerves actually have _____ within the muscle.

receptors

---

4. Sensory fibers which compose the muscle nerves range in size from _____ to _____.

I-IV
or
A-C

5. The types of receptors that have been identified for the remaining one-third of sensory fibers are mostly free nerve endings and a few Pacinian and paciniform corpuscles.

The roles of these receptors and the adequate stimuli necessary to activate them are not well understood. Most research with such endings involves electrical stimulation of the muscle nerves.

Electrical stimulation is not a functional or physiological input, and, therefore, may lead to confusion or misinterpretation of an activity under physiological conditions.

The majority of sensory receptors which have been identified in nerves supplying muscle are _____ _____ endings.

free nerve

---

6. There are a few Pacinian and _____ corpuscles.

paciniform

---

7. Pacinian corpuscles are generally served by fibers in the A-alpha (I) and A-beta (II) groups. The axons of paciniform corpuscles most likely belong to group A-beta (II) and _____ fibers.

A-delta (III)

---

8. It is apparent that these corpuscles respond to touch/pressure (Mountcastle, 1980). The endings that would activate the fastest axons would be the _____ corpuscles.

Pacinian

9. Pacinian and paciniform corpuscles respond to _____ stimuli.

touch/pressure

---

10. Free nerve endings arise from a wide range of axon diameters from groups A gamma-delta and C (II, III and IV). For many years, the prevailing thought concerning free nerve endings was that they were solely pain receptors (nociceptors). More recent evidence, however, shows them to be responsive to a variety of sensory modalities.

Of course, many of the free nerve endings do act as _____ receptors.

pain

---

11. Many of the unmeyelinated C (IV) fibers respond when the muscle is subjected to mild mechanical pressure of from 5 to 10 grams in intensity. Some C fibers respond to very light touch. Other such fibers may be activated by slight changes in temperature (Mendell and Henneman, 1980).

If the blood supply to the muscle is occluded by prolonged contraction, C fiber discharge is recorded and associated with the perception of _____.

pain

---

12. Free nerve endings which arise from unmeyelinated C fibers in muscle will respond to a variety of sensory stimuli including light _____, mild _____, and changes in _____.

touch
pressure
temperature

13. Many C (IV) fibers also act as nociceptors or _____ receptors.

pain

14. These C sensory fibers make polysynaptic connections with the _____ motor neurons.

alpha

15. The autonomic fibers which are found in muscle nerves are most likely vasomotor fibers and sympathetic fibers to the muscle spindle (Eldred, et.al., 1960). Vasomotor input controls the _____ _____.

blood vessels

16. When electrically stimulated, many of the afferent fibers smaller than group A-alpha (I) size produce activity in polysnaptic circuits which predominately result in excitation to flexors and _____ to _____.

inhibition
extensors

17. It could be assumed that all the mentioned stimuli would have the net effect of exciting _____ and inhibiting _____.

flexors
extensors

292

physiological

18. It must be remembered, however, that results from electrical stimulation may not completely parallel results from _____ activation.

19. It is still likely that stimulating the C fibers will result in eliciting the flexor reflexes. When engaged in patient treatment, the therapist should be cognizant of what stimuli are being applied to any muscle and the skin overlying it.

Responses, either desired or undesired, may result from the application of touch, pressure, pain or _____ to a muscle.

temperature

20. When handling a patient input other than stretch is undoubtedly impossible to avoid. The net effects of such input, however, must be considered.

You can gain insight into such effects on a patient by careful _____ of the patient.

observation

21. It is possible to capitalize upon these sensory effects by purposeful application of such stimuli and observation of the patient's _____.

response

22. Remember that the multisynaptic nature of small fiber connections results in prolonged activity. Once a response is elicited it may _____.

persist or continue

SUMMARY

The diagram shows the wide variety of fibers that may be found in nerves which innervate skeletal muscle.

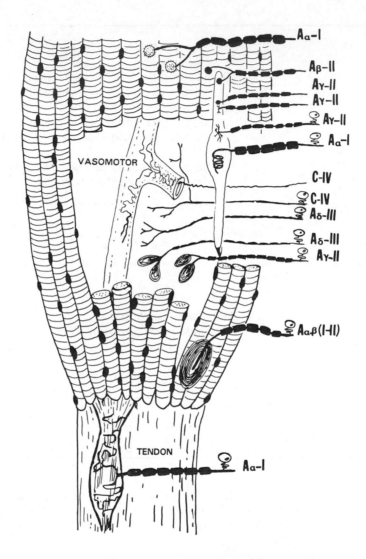

Activation of fibers that are smaller than A-alpha fibers may have the net affect of exciting flexor and inhibiting extensor muscles. When handling a patient some activation of such fibers is impossible to avoid. The response of the patient should be carefully monitored and the therapist should be aware of the stimuli being presented to the patient that is both desirable and undesirable.

Remember that the multisynaptic nature of small fiber connections result in prolonged activity. Once a response is elicited it may persist.

23. There are articular nerves which supply the joints and associated structures, just as there are muscle nerves which supply muscles.

   Just as with muscle nerves, the axons within the articular nerves represent a wide range of sizes from I to _____.

IV

---

24. It has been estimated that 45 percent of the fibers in articular nerves are A-gamma (II). Another 45 percent are C (IV) fibers , and 10 percent are large axons of the A-alpha (I) variety (Wyke, 1972).

   The greatest numbers of axons present in articular nerves are from groups _____ and _____.

A-gamma (II)
C (IV)

---

25. Unfortunately, for our clarity in identification of **joint receptors** as opposed to the **axons** which serve them, joint receptors have also been classified with a Roman numeral system. There are four types of joint receptors. These receptors are, therefore, classified as types I, _____, _____ and _____ (Wyke, 1972).

II, III, IV

---

26. Type I, II and III joint receptors are all encapsulated and are served by myelinated axons. Type IV receptors terminate in free nerve endings and are served by thinly myelinated _____.

axons

27. Joint receptors may also be placed in two broad categories: rapidly adapting and slowly adapting.

This categorization is also true of all _____.

receptors

28. Joints contain receptors of both the rapidly adapting and slowly adapting variety. These receptors also have a range from low threshold of activation to _____ _____ of activation.

high threshold

29. Because of the variety of responsiveness in joint receptors, it could be reasonable to assume a wide variety of conditions may be recorded by these _____ receptors.

joint

30. Type I joint receptors have been called Ruffini, or Ruffini-like, corpuscles. A type I joint receptor consists of a cluster of corpuscles. As the axon branch enters the corpuscle it looses its myelin and forms multiple branches of terminal endings.

Label the diagram.

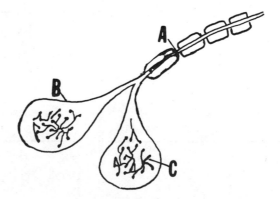

TYPE I JOINT RECEPTOR

a) axon
b) corpuscle
c) receptor endings

31. Type I joint receptors are slowly adapting mechano-receptors and have a low threshold of activation. These receptors are active **both** during movement and at rest.

    The type I joint receptors, therefore, have both static and _____ functions.

dynamic

_____

32. Because these joint receptors have a resting discharge they would be considered _____.

static

_____

33. Conditions which alter type I firing rates are joint movement, altered joint pressure and muscle contraction. Responsiveness to these modalities illustrate the receptor's _____ capability.

dynamic

_____

34. Type I joint receptors are: _____ adapting, _____ threshold receptors.

slowly
low

_____

35. Type I joint receptors serve both static and dynamic functions as they are active both at _____ and with _____.

rest
movement

36. Type I joint receptors are found in the ligaments and fibrous part of the joint capsule. They are more numerous in the proximal joints.

There would be a greater density of type I receptors in the knee joint than would be found in the _____ joint.

ankle

37. Type I joint receptors are served primarily by group A beta-gamma (II) afferent fibers. These receptors are acti-vated by muscle _____, and joint _____.

contraction
movement

38. Type I joint receptors are also activated by altera-tions in joint _____.

pressure

39. Type II joint receptors are referred to as having paciniform endings. The corpuscle contains a lami-nated, "onion-like" bulbous covering over the unmye-linated process within.

Type II receptors are rapidly adapting and have a low threshold for activation.

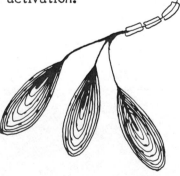

TYPE II JOINT RECEPTOR

Type I receptors are _____ adapting.

slowly

40. Type II receptors have _____ thresholds and are _____ adapting.

low
rapidly

_____

41. Type II receptors are active at the beginning and end of a movement.

Type I receptors are active _____ a movement.

during

_____

42. The paciniform receptors are located in the joint capsule at the synovial junction, and within the fat pads associated with the joint.

There are more type II receptors in the distal joints. Type I receptors have been reported to be more numerous in the _____ joints.

proximal

_____

43. When joint movement occurs, type II receptors are active at the _____ and _____ of the movement.

beginning or onset
end or termination

_____

44. There would be a greater density of type II receptors in the knee than there would be in the _____ joint.

hip

45. Both type I and II joint receptors are mechanoreceptors. Apparently movement produces a deformation of the capsule which produces generator _____ in the terminals.

potentials

---

46. Both the type I and type II joint receptors have _____ thresholds.

low

---

47. Type III joint receptors appear to be identical to Golgi tendon organs. In this case, instead of tendons, they are found in ligaments. Although there is some variation according to species, these endings are found just about everywhere except the cervical region of the spine. In the extremities the receptors are located in the collateral ligaments.

Type III joint receptors are dynamic and are slowly adapting. They have a high _____ to activation.

threshold

TYPE III JOINT RECEPTOR

---

48. Type III endings are not active in immobile joints. They are active only in the extreme ranges of joint movement either active or passive. They also respond to strong longitudinal traction.

Type III receptors are _____ adapting.

slowly

300

49. Type III joint receptors are active at the _____ of joint range.

extremes

50. An effective stimulus for activating type III receptors is longitudinal _____.

traction

51. Type III joint receptors are basically identical to the _____.

GTO

52. Type IV endings are not usually considered to be mechanoreceptors but rather pain receptors. They are located in joint ligaments, capsules and fat pads.

These receptors respond to extreme mechanical deformation of the joint and direct mechanical or chemical irritations. Most likely these nociceptors are similiar to those found in muscle (Hong, 1978).

Type IV receptors are served by group A-delta (III) and C (IV) afferent fibers and have _____ thresholds.

high

TYPE IV JOINT RECEPTOR

53. Type IV joint receptors terminate as _____ endings.

free

CLASSIFICATION OF JOINT RECEPTORS

TYPE	AXON CLASSIFICATION	RECEPTOR MORPHOLOGY	LOCATION IN JOINT	LOCATION IN BODY	THRESHOLD	ADAPTABILITY	FUNCTION
I	II	Ruffini-like	fibrous capsule and ligaments	proximal joints	low	slow	active at rest during movement
II	II	Paciniform	synovial junction of capsule, fat pads	distal joints	low	rapid	active at a beginning and end of movement
III	I	GTO-like	ligaments	all joints (except) cervical	high	slow	active at the extremes of range
IV	III-IV	Free nerve endings	ligaments, capsule fat pads	all joints	high	slow	active to extreme mechanical irritation and deformation

54. The functions of joint receptors are not fully understood. The information from research studies have come from animals with different types of experimental lesions. Work has been done on both normal humans and a variety of clinical patients. It is difficult to apply stimuli to an individual and be assured that only the system under study is activated.

Any contact with the skin (difficult to avoid) will influence the output from any associated or underlying system.

It is very difficult to isolate the effects of one type of _____ from another.

receptor

55. At one time, joint receptors were assumed to be solely responsible for kinesthesia. Kinesthesia is a term which is interpreted in a variety of ways. Actually the term means more than the ability to discriminate joint position. It includes discriminating the direction, amplitude and speed of movement as well as relative weight of body parts (Newton, 1982).

Recent experiments, particularly with patients who have had total joint replacements, have shown that joint position and movement sense persists in the absence of capsular sensory elements.

It is likely that an important role of joint receptors is to provide input to _____ centers.

higher

---

56. Just as with the muscle spindle and other muscle afferents, the most important role of joint receptors is most likely the information that is projected to _____ _____.

higher centers

---

57. Kinesthesia is a complex sense that depends on an integration of afferent information reaching the CNS over visual, vestibular, proprioceptive and somatic afferent systems (Mountcastle, 1980).

Among somatic contributions are joint receptors, muscle receptors and skin or cutaneous receptors. Alterations in any one of these systems does not appear to disturb kinesthesia functionally as long as other receptors are functioning.

Similarly, loss of the visual or vestibular systems does not destroy kinesthetic sense. Such loss may, however, distort the concept of body form and position.

Although a perceptual sense may not be destroyed by the loss of one type of sensory input, such a loss may result in perceptual _____.

distortion

303

58. Studies of the somatic systems suggest that normal performance of kinesthetic activity depends on the central integration of incoming signals from two or more **different** sets of peripheral afferent fibers.

The CNS apparently matches and compares information from the various sources and then decides which is valid. Lesions in the peripheral systems may produce a loss of or disturbances in kinesthesia.

Lesions in the cortex and other higher centers could also produce disturbances in _____.

kinesthesia

---

59. Because there is a distinct scheme of anatomical location and functional activation among the four types of joint receptors, hypotheses about their roles in movement control have often been postulated (Newton, 1982).

Again, we may consider the possible reflex responses that might occur from joint receptor input at the spinal level. Don't forget that the experimental literature is not complete and alternative answers may exist.

It has been stated that joint receptor activation has "profound effects on muscle tone" (Wyke, 1972). It has also been stated that spinal reflex initiated by joint receptors are not particularly powerful (Bishop, 1982).

There are conflicting reports in the literature concerning the function of _____ _____.

joint receptors

---

60. Joint receptors most likely do not make monosynaptic connections with motor neurons. They do, however, make spinal connections via the _____ pool.

interneuron

---

61. In general, these multisynaptic reflex circuits made with joint receptors tend to inhibit flexors and facilitate _____ (Bishop, 1982).

extensors

304

62. We usually think of sensory input as causing or facilitating motor output. With the muscle spindle, however, the motor activity enhances the output from the sensory receptors. Because of this relationship, activity in the fusimotor system can be inferred from observing sensory receptor output.

Studies which measure gamma motor output indirectly through recording activity from muscle spindle afferents show that application of pressure in the contralateral knee joint results in an increased output from triceps sural afferents (Appleberg, et.al., 1979).

Thus, joint receptor input affects the excitation level of _____ motor neurons.

gamma

---

63. According to Lundberg (1975), interneurons in the GTO pathways receive convergent excitation from low threshold cutaneous and joint afferents. Joint receptor input can, therefore, alter the reflex response of the GTO's.

Recording excitatory levels from anterior horn cells, joint receptor input was found to alter the inhibitory and excitatory pathways that originated with the _____.

GTO's

---

64. When intraarticular pressure is increased by saline injections in the knee joint of cats and man inhibition of extensors and facilitation of _____ was noted.

flexors

---

65. Obviously, joint afferent activation does not always result in excitation of the _____ muscles.

extensor

305

66. Joint receptors, like muscle receptors, appear to support muscular reflex activity. However, **no** peripheral input alone is responsible for "driving" motor neuron activity.

From a clinical point of view, this is neither discouraging nor unexpected news.

Reflex **support** may be all that is necessary in assisting the patient in producing or gaining control over a _____.

movement

---

67. If a patient has not moved, or has moved abnormally for a period of time, the normal input which results from correct movement is probably lacking.

As a result, the patient may no longer "know" how to _____.

move

---

68. Stimulating joint receptors through assisted movement and other techniques such as joint approximation and traction may provide lost _____ _____ to higher centers.

sensory input

---

69. Such stimulation which increases sensory receptor output may reflexly initiate or **assist** _____.

movement

---

70. Driving motor activity with peripheral receptors is not possible. Peripheral inputs may, however, help the patient by providing reflex _____ to the movement.

support or assistance

71. Almost everyone who has utilized manual therapy is likely to be familiar with the patient who presents with pain and muscle weakness. Upon examination, a joint displacement is identified and corrected. There is an immediate and dramatic change in muscle strength. Such a rapid change, therefore, could not be the result of an actual pathological change in the

_____.

muscle or
connective tissue

---

72. Wyke (1972) has described a wide range of receptors that are present in each synovial joint. These pain and mechanoreceptor afferents are found in the joint capsule, fat pads, and ligaments. The activation of these receptors is reported to have marked effects on muscle "tone."

Reflex inhibition of muscle could occur when joint displacement results in the stimulation of certain _____ _____.

joint receptors

---

73. According to Wyke (1979), type I receptors are the only joint afferents which project to the cortex for conscious awareness. These receptors play a powerful role in kinesthesia as well as in reflex generation. Types II through IV are primarily involved in the production of _____.

reflexes

---

74. Joint receptors provide sensory input to higher centers which is undoubtedly useful in motor learning sequences and other activities which require or are enhanced by kinesthetic input.

Joint receptors also have an effect on the state of muscle contraction from inputs at a _____ level.

spinal

307

75. Wyke has researched joint afferents for many years. Although some of his work has not been corroborated by other researchers, a partial explanation may be differences in research design. It would appear useful to explore his findings as they have direct clinical application. Keep in mind that some of this information may not be reliable. Most of the information in frames 74-108 is directly from Wyke.

As noted before, joint afferents are distributed differently in _____ than in _____ joints.

proximal
distal

---

76. According to Wyke, there are arthrostatic and arthro kinetic reflexes. The former relate to the discharge in stationary joints, the latter to the discharge in response to _____ _____.

joint movement

---

77. The differences in joint angle that can be detected in proximal joints is about 1.4 degrees whereas in the terminal interphalangeal joints it is about 10 degrees (Wyke, 1979).

It does appear foolish then to test a patient's general kinesthetic senses by picking up a hand or foot and instructing the patient to tell you if the finger or toe is up or down.

Early diagnosis of kinesthetic disturbances may depend on examining the most sensitive joints to detect the slightest disturbances. Problems should be more apparent and detected earlier in joints which are the most sensitive to changes in joint angles.

The most appropriate joints to examine for general kinesthetic awareness may be the _____ joints.

proximal

---

78. The ability to detect the direction of joint movement involves what has been described as _____ reflexes.

arthrokinetic

79. The mechanoreceptor population reaches its highest density in proximal joints. Conversely, the distal interphalangeal joints contain very few such receptors.

This distribution may be one reason why an individual's perceptual accuracy could be greater with the _____ limb joints than the _____ limb joints.

proximal
distal

---

80. General kinesthesia of the lower extremity may be best assessed at the _____ joint.

hip

---

81. The evaluation of **postural** sense is another matter. This cannot be accomplished by moving the joint but rather requires an awareness of static joint position and joint stresses such as when it is bearing body weight.

Thus, there are arthostatic reflexes and _____ reflexes.

arthrokinetic

---

82. According to Wyke, all these reflexes work together in complex patterns during normal movement and in achieving more postural activities such as standing or balancing on one foot.

For instance, passive manipulation of an isolated hip joint which is moved into abduction and held there, produces complex coordinated reflex changes in many muscles of the lower extremity as measured by electromyography.

The reflex activity not only appears in the muscles of the moving limb but in the contra-lateral limb as well.

These reflexes are excitatory in some instances and _____ in others.

inhibitory

83. If the joint that was abducted is reversed into adduction different responses occur because the pattern of stress on the joint capsule is different during the adduction movement than it was during the previous abduction movement.

The arrangement of the joint receptors may be different from one portion of the joint capsule to another.

Reciprocal movements such as abduction and adduction may produce entirely different _____ _____ _____.

joint receptor responses

---

84. Type III receptors (Golgi-like) are primarily inhibitory. If enough traction is applied to stimulate them, muscle activity is grossly _____.

inhibited

---

85. Pain resulting from the activation of nociceptive the joint receptors may cause reflex muscle contractions or spasm.

Alleviation of this type of joint input will result in muscle _____.

relaxation

---

86. Standing and weight-shifting and other such activities involve different patterns of joint stress and joint movement than does moving a non-weight-bearing extremity through an arc of movement.

These postural responses involve coordination of the _____ reflexes.

arthostatic

---

87. There is a greater population of type I joint receptors in the _____ joints.

proximal

II

The distal joints contain the major concentration of type _____ receptors.

88. Evaluation of the arthrostatic reflexes or postural sense can be done with a set of posture testing materials such as a screen with a vertical line painted on it which is perpendicular to the floor.

The vertical line is the true axis. Have the patient stand so that the body axis is in line with the true axis.

Ask the patient to stand on one foot and then the other with eyes closed to eliminate visual righting reactions.

If a series of photographs are taken, it is possible to measure the angles between the body axes and true axis which would be a measure of the deviation from _____.

normal

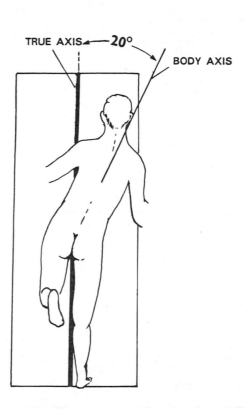

89. In the diagram above the deviation from vertical is _____ degrees.

90. You should undoubtedly find a range of normal responses for **your** laboratory setup and procedure. Wyke has suggested +/- 1½° from the vertical is a normal range.

    This procedure should provide an assessment of _____ sense.

arthrostatic
or
postural

NOTE: Other proprioceptors such as the vestibular apparatus and the muscle spindle and exteroceptors also contribute to position sense.

---

91. Joint mechanoreceptors can be injured or destroyed by trauma, disease or immobilization.

    An athlete who had a severe ankle sprain may recover and appear normal until a real demand is placed on that ankle such as walking in the dark or in an athletic event.

    When tested for postural sense under the above conditions, he may show marked postural deviation when he is standing on the _____ _____.

involved ankle

---

92. From such mechanoreceptor loss the posture of the whole body may be altered. A careful analysis of walking and running would most likely show abnormalities as well.

    Mechanoreceptors may be injured or destroyed by _____, _____, and _____.

trauma
disease
immobilization

---

93. A patient may have a long leg cast applied to the lower extremity because of a fractured femur.

    This treatment may cause problems at both the knee and ankle joints because of _____.

immobilization

94. Treatment for such loss or injury may include the use of a balance board. These are available commercially but one can be made from a round or oval piece of wood which acts as a platform. Half a wooden ball is attached on the underside so that it is unstable in all directions.

Exercising with this rockerboard may promote vestibular reflexes, stretch reflexes and joint reflexes as the body attempts to compensate for the joint that is injured. The rockerboard may also help activate any remaining intact receptors and stimulate regeneration of those which were lost.

Don't expect immediate miracles. It may take months to achieve _____ _____.

normal function

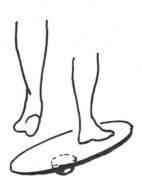

95. In a personal communication with colleagues Wyke has explained the mechanism by which stress or the lack of it affects the joint receptors.

The capsule develops around the nerve ending in response to stress. The capillaries then grow around the capsule in response to its presence. When the everyday stresses upon the joint receptor structures is lacking the structures will degenerate.

Exercising with a rockerboard or a similar device could provide the necessary stresses to stimulate regeneration of lost or damaged _____ _____.

joint receptors

96. Patients with involvement of one hip joint, as with monoarticular rheumatoid arthritis may show less vertical deviation but will likely show more abnormal posturing of the lower extremities.

According to Wyke the input from the hip may have a more bilateral distribution than does input from the ankle. Loss at one hip, therefore, may be more apparent bilaterally than is loss at one ankle.

There are likely to be postural abnormalities with loss of _____ _____.

joint receptors

---

97. Postural responses are not totally abolished with mechanoreceptor loss. The observation that residual function remains after total joint replacement attests to that fact. It is quite likely, however, that there are subtle or even not so subtle alterations in postural responses.

Such abnormalities might not be apparent until the individual tries to move about in the dark or perhaps puts the joint under stress such as stepping up or down in a precarious activity with the involved _____.

extremity

---

98. Some clinicians have indicated to the authors that the joint replacement patient may do very well with one replacement such as the hip. When more than one joint is replaced, such as both the hip and ankle, postural responses are highly compromised.

These observations would suggest that the receptors in one joint assist in providing sensory feedback which may relate to another _____.

joint

---

99. Multiple joint replacements may markedly compromise _____ response.

postural

100. Wyke indicates that some surgeons are attempting to leave intact as much of the joint capsule as possible during total joint surgery. He suggests that patients receiving such surgery have less postural abnormalities than those who do not.

With mechanoreceptor loss, postural responses are not totally _____.

abolished

---

101. If it is true that joint receptors degenerate during immobilization, care should be taken to limit the number of joints involved and the length of time of immobilization. Isometric exercises will help maintain joint receptors as the muscle tension produces a deformation of the joint capsule.

When immobilization is terminated special care should be taken to evaluate and treat possible loss of _____ and _____ reflexes.

arthrokinetic
arthrostatic

---

102. The aging process results in a decrease of mechanoreceptors as well as other types of receptors. This loss may in part account for the susceptibility of the elderly to fall frequently.

Such receptor loss may also contribute to the decrease in discriminatory abilities of the _____ patient.

elderly

315

103. In conditions of spasticity in which there is increased tension from muscles crossing the joint, the output from joint receptors will be augmented. If spastic joints are immobile or relatively so, disturbances in mechanoreceptors might also be expected.

In these situations, appropriate rehabilitation measures should be directed to the _____.

joints

---

104. Evidence suggests that mechanoreceptors have input onto gamma motor neurons. It has been observed that changes in tendon jerks occur in situations where there is articular pathology.

Of course, augmented background input to the alpha motor neurons and a concurrent stretch input could also result in increased _____ _____ reflexes.

tendon jerk

---

105. According to Wyke, the slowly adapting mechanoreceptors project to type I motor units and rapidly adapting mechanoreceptors project to type _____ units.

II

---

106. If this is the case, type I joint receptors at least would contribute to the postural influences of type _____ motor units.

I

---

107. Movement and weight bearing of the proximal joints should augment these _____ functions.

postural

108. Wyke strongly recommends the use of a rocking chair to produce rhythmical stimulation of muscle spindles and all the articular mechanoreceptors in the joints of the lumbar spine and the hips, knees and ankles. Such activity also produces rhythmical stimulation of the mechanoreceptors on the skin that is being stretched and restretched by movements of the joints.

The rocking chair activity may diminish pain in the lower body through this mechanism. It is also an exercise, of a partially weight bearing nature, that should be excellent for the elderly almost irrespective of their physical condition.

Such activity would provide excellent vestibular stimulation as well. (See Barnes, Crutchfield, and Heriza, **The Neurophysiological Basis of Patient Treatment, Vol. IV— The Vestibular System**)

Rocking chair activities may diminish the loss of mechanoreceptors in an elderly patient who might otherwise be _____.

immobilized

SUMMARY

Nerve fibers present in articular nerves vary in size from A to C. Joint receptors supplied by these axons have been classified into four types: I, II, III and IV (see chart on page 302). Many of these receptors are mechanoreceptors.

Type I: These receptors are more numerous in the proximal joints. They are active both during movement and at rest. They are low threshold and slowly adapting.

Type II: These receptors are more numerous in the distal joints. They are active at the beginning and end of movements. They are low threshold and rapidly adapting.

Type III: These receptors are indistinguishable from GTO's. They are not active in immobile joints and are active only at the extreme limits of joint range. They have high thresholds and are slowly adapting.

Type IV: These receptors are pain receptors.

The functions of joint receptors and their possible contributions to muscular reflexes and kinesthesia are difficult to evaluate, and conflicting evidence as to their roles persists in the literature.

Much of the clinical application presented in this section is based upon the observations and opinions of Barry Wyke. It must be kept in mind that not all of his work has been corroborated, and some of this material may not be completely reliable. As therapists we can apply these observations to our patients, keeping in mind that responses should be carefully monitored and that through our own clinical observations and research the information may be clarified.

Activation of joint receptors results in modification of the state of muscle contraction. Whether this response is weak or powerful has been debated by investigators. One clinical example which tends to support the effect of joint receptors on muscle contraction is the situation in which the patient presents with pain and weakness and a joint displacement is also found to be present. If the joint displacement is corrected there is an immediate and dramatic change in muscle strength. This rapid change could only be reflex based and logically would seem to be a direct result of alteration in joint receptor output.

In general, the reflex circuits in which joint receptors participate tend to provide excitation to extensor muscles and inhibition to flexor muscles.

Joint receptors provide input to reflex circuits which alters the output of other receptors such as the spindle afferents and the GTO.

According to Wyke, there are arthrostatic reflexes (stationary joints and postural sense) and arthrokinetic reflexes which relate to moving joints.

Testing joint position sense is probably best evaluated by testing the proximal joints. These joints are reported to detect differences in joint angle as small as 1.4 degrees. The distal joints will detect differences no less than 10 degrees.

The evaluation of postural sense requires weight bearing or static joint positioning. Thus, these arthrostatic reflexes can be evaluated using postural testing materials. Balance boards and rocking chairs provide some avenues for treatment of impaired kinesthetic sense and postural reflexes.

The contribution of joint receptors to kinesthetic sense is difficult to evaluate as other sensory systems cannot be eliminated during testing. It is generally believed that most peripheral receptors (muscle, tendon, vestibular, visual, cutaneous and joint receptors) contribute to kinesthesia. Loss of one system does not appear to greatly impair this sense. Loss of or alterations in multiple systems, however, create appreciable deficits.

As with other peripheral receptors, the greatest or most important contribution of joint receptor input may be through the projections to higher centers.

109. A discussion of pheripheral influences on muscle activity would not be complete without considering receptors which are located in the skin. The skin is the largest organ system in the body and it is richly supplied with sensory endings.

Stimulation of body tissues results in five different qualities of sensation. These are touch/pressure, cold, warmth, pain and kinesthesia. The latter we have already discussed. The first four are most highly developed in the skin.

If you consider that all muscles and joints are covered by skin, it is easy to recognize that cutaneous inputs may also have regulatory effects on _____.

muscle

---

110. The following is an illustration of a section of skin.

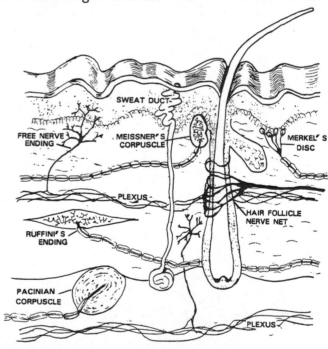

Meissner's
Ruffini
Pacinian
Merkel's

Examples of incapsulated endings are _____, _____, _____ corpuscles and _____ discs.

111. The following receptors have been identified in glabrous (non-hairy) skin.

RECEPTORS IN GLABROUS OR NON-HAIRY SKIN

Receptor	Modality		Fiber Type
Merkel's discs	Mechanoreceptor	Touch/pressure	A-beta
Meissner's corpuscles	Mechanoreceptor	Contact & vibration	A-beta
Pacinian corpuscles	Mechanoreceptor	Contact & vibration	A-beta
Free nerve ending	Thermoreceptor	Cold	A-delta
Free nerve ending	Nociceptor	Prickling pain/tickle	A-delta
Free nerve ending	Thermoreceptor	Warmth	C
Free nerve ending	Nociceptor	Burning pain/itch	C

Free nerve endings in non-hairy skin have axons in both _____ and _____ groups.

A or III
C or IV

112. The three mechanoreceptors serve different qualities of touch-pressure and flutter-vibration.

The Merkel's discs are velocity and position detectors and provide a sense of **touch-pressure**.

The Meissner's corpuscles are velocity detectors and provide a sense of **contact** and **flutter** (low frequency).

The Pacinian corpuscles are velocity and perhaps position detectors. They provide a sense of contact and **vibration** (high frequency).

These mechanoreceptors are all served by type _____ afferent fibers.

A beta (II)

113. Free nerve endings are served by both A-_____ and _____ fibers.

delta (III)
C (IV)

321

114. In non-hairy skin the free nerve endings with the A-delta are either thermoreceptors or nociceptors. The same division occurs in free nerve endings served by C fibers.

The thermoreceptors with the A-delta fibers provide a sense of **cooling**. The C fiber type provide a sense of **warming** (Mountcastle, 1980).

Free nerve endings that are thermoreceptors serve both the senses of _____ and _____.

heat
cold

115. Warming is a sense mediated by _____ fiber receptors.

C

116. Cooling is a sense mediated by _____ fiber receptors.

A-delta

117. The fast-conducting fibers serve nociceptors which provide the sense of **prickling pain** at high frequencies. At low frequencies, we experience **tickle** through these fibers.

These nociceptors are served by type _____ fibers.

A-delta

118. The C fibers serve nociceptors that provide at high frequencies a sense of **burning pain** and at low frequencies, **itch**.

These receptors are _____ nerve endings.

free

119. In hairy skin there are some differences. The A-beta fiber group of axons serve 3 different receptors in hairy skin:

RECEPTORS IN HAIRY SKIN

Receptor	Modality		Fiber Type
Hair follicle net	Mechanoreceptor	Contact & flutter	A-beta
Free nerve ending	Mechanoreceptor	Contact	A-beta
Ruffini organs	Mechanoreceptor	Touch/pressure	A-beta
Pacinian corpuscles	Mechanoreceptor	Velocity/position & vibration	A-beta
Free nerve ending	Thermoreceptor	Warmth	C
Free nerve ending	Nociceptor	Burning pain/itch	C

Also present are the A-beta type Pacinian corpuscles which provide a sense of _____ and _____.

contact
vibration

---

120. The hair follicle apparatus provides a sense of **contact** and **flutter** in hairy skin. Meissner's corpuscles are responsible for these senses in _____ skin.

non-hairy

---

121. The free nerve endings served by the fast A-beta fibers provide a sense of **contact**. The Ruffini organs provide the sense of **touch-pressure**.

In non-hairy skin the latter sense is the responsibility of the _____ _____.

Merkel's Discs

---

122. The cutaneous input is also most important in that it relays to higher centers for _____ _____.

conscious awareness

323

123. The deep tissues such as fascia have sparse mechanorecptor innervation and those afferents have high thresholds. If the skin is anesthetized the threshold to detection of pressure is increased several times.

Pacinian corpuscles are abundant in interosseus membranes and near the bone. As a result we are exquisitely sensitive to vibration in deep tissues.

There appears to be a significant nociceptive (pain) innervation to fascia and other deep tissues.

Two modalities that will be perceived in deep tissues are _____ and _____.

vibration
pain

---

124. Cutaneous receptors also exert spinal reflex influences through inputs to spinal _____.

interneurons

---

125. These receptors provide feedback for orientation to the environment and for protection. The most likely responses resulting from cutaneous stimulation are flexor withdrawal responses.

Flexor reflexes are inhibitory to _____ muscles.

extensor

---

126. Stimulation of certain areas of the skin such as the ball of the foot result in extension reflexes which assist in weight bearing.

Not all cutaneous input, therefore, inhibits _____ muscles.

extensor

127. In hairy skin there are also mechanoreceptors which are free nerve endings served by the A-delta fibers. They provide a sense of **contact.**

The A-delta (III) or C (IV) fiber free nerve endings which are thermoreceptors and nociceptors are the same as those in _____ skin.

non-hairy

---

128. Afferent fibers of different sizes are distributed in different proportions in different nerves. The ratio of C to A fibers may be 5:1 in nerves innervating proximal structures. In the face and hand there are much larger numbers of A fibers and the ratio of A to C fibers is approximately 1:1 (Mountcastle, 1980).

Those body areas which have the greatest requirement for acute sensitivity have the greatest number of _____ fibers.

myelinated or A

---

129. Although fiber classes of different sizes serve different sensory functions there is a great overlap in size and function. Therefore, the size and conduction velocity does not divide fibers by modality.

All input from a single modality is not carried in the same _____ axon.

size

---

130. Areas of the body which are served by fast conducting axons with exquisite power of discrimination are the _____ and _____.

face
hand

325

131. It is clear to most clinicians that the state of awareness or excitability of the patient has definite effects on the patient's response to sensory input.

Physiologists have been aware that certain reactions occur which affect sensory perception. For example, visual acuity is affected by autonomic adjustments of the pupil of the eye.

It is now apparent that most, if not all, sensory receptors such as the muscle spindle, cutaneous receptors and joint mechanoreceptors receive an **autonomic** innervation.

Such autonomic activity may alter the sensitivity of receptors and affect the receptor's _____ (Mountcastle, 1980).

response

---

132. Most if not all sensory receptors receive innervation from the _____ _____ system.

autonomic nervous

---

133. An interesting clinical case was observed by a colleague who was evaluating a patient in a pain clinic (Cummings, 1984). The patient had very specific pain in joints of the hand. This patient did not respond to therapeutic intervention for her pain. A stellate ganglion block was performed and the pain disappeared.

The autonomic input to the patient joint receptors may have augmented or even perpetrated her perception of joint _____.

pain

---

134. Sympathetic nervous system input to mechano-receptors lower the threshold of activation and slows adaptation to stimuli. The presence of epinephrine produces the same effect.

These inputs cause in increase in the generator potential _____.

amplitude

326

135. Some of the unmyelinated fibers which supply muscle spindles are apparently sympathetic fibers. Repetitive stimulation of these autonomic motor fibers increases the discharge rate of the afferent receptors.

Sympathetic input to receptors could increase the magnitude of reflex _____.

responses

---

136. If an individual is excited, angry or in pain, there is increased output from the sympathetic nervous system.

Such system activation would include an increased autonomic stimulation to numerous _____ _____.

sensory receptors

---

137. Once again consider the chart in which peripheral fibers are classified. It is useful at this time to add some additional information. (Use chart to answer questions 137-140)

Dorsal Root Fibers	Ventral Root Fibers	Conduction Velocities (a function of axon diameter)	Nature of Synaptic Networks
I	A-alpha	75-120 m/sec	Monosynaptic
II	A-beta-gamma	35-75 m/sec	↑
III	A-delta	5-30 m/sec	
	B	3-15 m/sec	↓
IV	C	.05-2 m/sec	Polysynaptic

As noted before, different modalities such as touch, pressure and temperature are served by axons of _____ sizes.

all (or most)

138. The larger fibers tend to make more _____ synaptic connections.

mono

139. The activation of C fibers initiates action in a _____-synaptic network.

poly

140. If you wish a more localized, specific, controlled response, the fibers that would be the most likely to do that are _____.

A-alpha

141. Remember, there may be as many as 5 times the number of C fibers in relation to A fibers. If you wish more diffuse, generalized and prolonged response with less control, a likely candidate for activation may be the _____ fiber.

C

142. It has been noted that A and C·fibers have different recovery patterns.

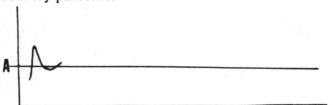

The C fiber has a prolonged after-hyperpolarization or positive after potential. This quality should make it more difficult to re-activate than an _____ fiber.

A

143. Neurophysiologists have noted that a fast-repetitive stimulus applied to a C fiber will result in a change of the positive after-potential to a negative after-potential. Application of such a stimulus should make it easier to activate the _____ fiber (Mountcastle, 1980; Johnson, 1980).

C

---

144. The concept of "brushing" presented by Margaret Rood, OT, PT, was based on this information. **If** there were 5 times as many cutaneous C fibers than A; and **if** they could be made responsive by fast-repetitive input; and **if** their responses could be prolonged because of the highly polysynaptic nature of their connections--**then** a technique which would activate them should "stir things up" and produce some affect on the motor neurons.

With such increased sensory input one might well expect increased _____ _____.

motor output

---

145. Of course, you would apply the sensory input to the cutaneous dermatomes that correspond to the innervation levels of the muscle that you wish to _____ (Hagbarth, 1952).

activate

---

146. There are inherent difficulties with such technqiues. First, the very diffuse nature of the response makes it difficult to evaluate the appropriateness, desirability or effectiveness of the technique.

As the technique works only sometimes but not invariably, most clinicians find that the response is too _____.

variable

147. We also know that the greatest excitation from cutaneous input is to the type IIB motor units and the dynamic gamma motor neurons. The **original** goal of brushing was to facilitate stability through tonic alpha and gamma responses. Obviously, it may not be possible to do that with cutaneous input.

Furthermore, in a particular patient it may not be desirable to preferentially recruit type _____ motor units.

II

---

148. Cutaneous input also produces the strongest response in _____ gamma neurons.

dynamic

---

149. You will recall that cutaneous fiber inputs tend to produce a net effect of excitation of flexors and inhibition of _____.

extensors

---

150. This pattern most likely occurs because reflexes are protective in nature. If threatened, the organism can withdraw or curl up. This withdrawal is usually a rapid movement and as such may involve the type _____ motor units.

II

---

151. So you can see that the cutaneous pathways favor the elicitation of withdrawal or _____ reflexes.

flexor
or
protective

152. Individuals who already have a high central "gain," or who have deficits in central integration or who are in a hyperexcitable state may produce marked defensive or withdrawal responses to exteroceptive stimuli. Often as therapists we call these individuals "tactile defensives."

Brief cutaneous stimulation in particular is most likely to elicit _____ reflexes.

flexor or
withdrawal or
protective

_____

153. Melzack and Wall (1965) promulgated the "gate control" theory of pain. In this theory, it is postulated that incoming impulses enter the cord and project to an area called the substantia gelatinosa. There are inhibitory interneurons in this area which control the input to second order neurons.

Large fiber input excites the interneurons so that input is decreased (closes the gate) and small fiber input inhibits the interneuron, the net effect of which is to decrease inhibition in second order neurons (opens the gate).

This theory has been challenged and modified overtime but has not been refuted. It is also only a partial explanation of sensory modulation. Nevertheless, it may be useful to consider application of this information.

One way to decrease central excitatory inputs from C fibers would be to excite _____ fibers.

A or large

_____

154. The largest fiber supplying a receptor in the skin is the A-beta axon from the Pacinian corpuscle. It may be possible, therefore, to inhibit adversive cutaneous input (or avoid it altogether) by slowly applying firm _____ to the skin.

pressure

155. As most of the cutaneous receptors are of the rapidly-adapting variety, a maintained stimulus such as pressure over a large area will eventually fail to stimulate these receptors because they require repetitive activation.

In this case, the excessive input from the rapidly adapting receptors could not continue to bombard the spinal circuits.

When attempting to "desensitize" or normalize the reaction to sensory input we might wish to decrease the activation of rapidly-adapting receptors. Stimulus application, therefore, should be firm, slow and _____.

maintained

---

156. When attempting to desensitize the patient's reaction to sensory stimuli, it is helpful to apply the stimuli over a broad area, such as using two hands to produce firm, maintained touch or pressure.

Maintaining pressure over an area prevents other forms of stimuli from reaching the other cutaneous _____ in that area.

receptors

---

157. If, on the other hand, you wish to "stir things up" and stimulate movement, you should apply stimuli lightly and quickly. Try it on yourself. This technique has an "irritating" quality and you tend to move in response to it.

The major drawback is that you are most likely to facilitate _____ responses or reflexes.

flexor or
withdrawal or
protective

---

158. An excellent technique for desensitizing areas is vibration. Remember that vibration can be used as a proprioceptive stimulus to elicit the tonic vibration reflex which produces _____ contraction.

muscle

159. A vibrator applied lightly to the skin over a broad area excites a different receptor than when applied to the muscle. In the latter case vibration stimulates the muscle spindle. Which of the cutaneous receptors is responsible for the sense of vibration? _____ _____.

Pacinian corpuscle

---

160. According to Sato and Ozaki (1966) if the Pacinian corpuscle is repetitively stimulated by vibration, it will supress other information from that area of the skin. Perhaps this is a further example of the gate mechanism. Perhaps there is an extensive pre-synaptic input from Pacinian corpuscles to other cutaneous afferents.

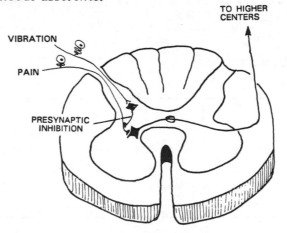

Try this on yourself if you are ticklish (or on someone else if you are not). Tickle the bottom of your foot and notice the sensations or response. Now apply a vibrator for 30 seconds or so. Tickle again. Notice any difference in sensitivity?

Vibratory input will usually supress sensitivity to other _____ inputs.

cutaneous

---

161. Sensitivity to various types of cutaneous stimuli can be suppressed through the use of _____.

vibration

162. Have you ever operated a chain-saw or other such device that produces heavy vibration to the hands? If so, after prolonged use you may have noticed that your control over hand movements is impaired and your hands feel numb.

These observations suggest that sensory input may be altered with _____.

vibration

---

163. According to Wyke (1979) the application of vibration to an appropriate area of the skin will result in blocking of pain inputs for up to several hours. He postulates this mechanism to be one of pre-synaptic inhibition on incoming pain afferents by the _____ _____.

Pacinian corpuscle

---

164. The motor unit type which is most susceptible to inhibition from cutaneous input is the type _____.

I

---

165. Manual contact with a patient can hardly be avoided. In fact, manual contact is an integral part of most techniques.

To avoid facilitating withdrawal reactions, manual contacts should be _____ and _____.

firm
maintained

---

166. The therapist should also be careful **where** the manual contact occurs.

If you do not wish to facilitate the biceps muscle, do not contact the skin over the _____ muscle.

biceps

167. Rothstein (1982) has raised a valid question concerning the facilitation of muscle contraction through cutaneous and proprioceptive input during exercise. We do not know whether the facilitated patterns of muscle recruitment and contraction ever resemble those of a "normal" contraction in functional situations. If some input or manipulation is necessary to initiate movement, however, it may not matter that the input is not completely appropriate.

Therapists should always question their actions and evaluate the treatment outcome through careful _____ of patient responses.

observation

---

168. Muscle is, indeed, mutable tissue. It undergoes profound changes when its pattern of use is altered or in the presence of disease. It is just as likely that therapeutic intervention can produce desirable changes or prevent undesirable ones from occuring.

Any avenue through which such influences can be effected is worth attempting, studying, questioning and researching.

We have many questions in terms of rehabilitating the patient with spasticity. Application of stretch or other such attention to the spastic muscle could result in extra input to an already augmented defect in central reflex gain. Such input may produce an excessive _____ _____.

motor output

---

169. On the other hand, experiments with stretch applied under certain conditions have shown a decrease in spacticity. The way in which the stretch is performed substantially determines the response. In addition, patients have different lesions which modify the response to stretch stimuli.

It is logical that patients will react differently to individual _____ programs.

treatment

335

170. Margaret Johnstone (1983) recommends the use of plastic inflatable air splints on spastic extremities to reduce the effects of spasticity.

A research project was carried out in her center, utilizing EMG recordings. EMG tracings were made from both flexors and extensors as forceful movements were made against the spastic wrist flexors. Marked clonic responses were noted and flexor activity persisted between stretches.

An air pressure splint was applied to the extremity which was then immobilized in a "reflex inhibiting recovery pattern" for 1 hour. There was a marked decrease in EMG activity to passive wrist extension.

This experiment most likely illustrates the result of decreasing afferent traffic onto the _____ _____.

motor neurons

---

171. The air splints are inflated by mouth. The breath consists of warm moist air and, when inflated, the splints provide a steady and equal pressure over the entire extremity. No sensory receptors should be activated except perhaps pressure receptors. These will adapt rapidly and even this traffic will cease.

A decrease in afferent input to the motor neuron and interneuron pools should result in a decrease in _____.

spasticity
or
motor neuron output

---

172. Of course, maintainence of the extremity in the splint prevents stretch and other input from influencing the extremity while more proximal parts are manipulated.

Constant pressure over the extremity decreases the input from a multitude of _____ receptors.

cutaneous

336

173. Inflatable splints completely cover the extremity providing a barrier from outside stimulation.

In addition, the constant pressure will likely inhibit small fiber input and then the pressure receptors themselves will _____.

adapt

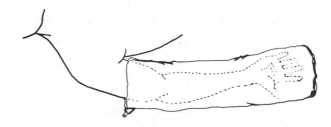

---

174. Margaret Johnstone (1983) states that "no amount of treatment is successful in many cases if spasticity is not attacked twenty-four hours a day by using inhibiting patterns or positioning."

Treatment which is given twenty-four hours a day may prevent or alter the structural and functional changes which contribute to spasticity, therefore, controlling the development of _____ itself.

spasticity

---

175. A most important part of Johnstone's statement is "... by using inhibiting patterns or positioning". Peripheral input, or the suppression of peripheral input may assist your treatment but it is not everything.

Patterns of movement must be changed. Most, if not all, treatment approaches involve movement re-_____.

education

337

SUMMARY

Cutaneous receptors primarily mediate the senses of touch/pressure, cold, warmth and pain.   There are several specific receptors which mediate these senses.

RECEPTORS IN GLABROUS OR NON-HAIRY SKIN

Receptor	Modality		Fiber Type
Merkel's discs	Mechanoreceptor	Touch/pressure	A-beta
Meissner's corpuscles	Mechanoreceptor	Contact & vibration	A-beta
Pacinian corpuscles	Mechanoreceptor	Contact & vibration	A-beta
Free nerve ending	Thermoreceptor	Cold	A-delta
Free nerve ending	Nociceptor	Prickling pain/tickle	A-delta
Free nerve ending	Thermoreceptor	Warmth	C
Free nerve ending	Nociceptor	Burning pain/itch	C

RECEPTORS IN HAIRY SKIN

Receptor	Modality		Fiber Type
Hair follicle net	Mechanoreceptor	Contact & flutter	A-beta
Free nerve ending	Mechanoreceptor	Contact	A-beta
Ruffini organs	Mechanoreceptor	Touch/pressure	A-beta
Pacinian corpuscles	Mechanoreceptor	Velocity/position & vibration	A-beta
Free nerve ending	Thermoreceptor	Warmth	C
Free nerve ending	Nociceptor	Burning pain/itch	C

Cutaneous receptors exert influence over muscle contraction through spinal stimulus/response circuits.   Cutaneous input may provide excitation to either the flexor or extensor muscles. The net effect of most cutaneous stimulation, however, is in favor of the flexor muscle groups.   These receptors are usually referred to as flexor reflex afferents (FRA's).

Afferent fibers of different sizes are distributed in different proportions to specific areas.   For example, the rates of C to A fibers on the proximal structures is 5:1, whereas in the face and hands (high discriminatory requirement) the ratio may be 1:1.

All sensory receptors apparently receive input from the autonomic nervous system. Sympathetic input to the receptor lowers the threshold of activation and slows its adaption to stimuli. This sympathetic nervous system input augments the receptor response.

Small, slow C fibers tend to participate in highly polysynaptic reflex circuits. If therapeutic sensory input activates these fibers the results may be prolonged, diffuse and variable.

The circuits involving A fibers tend to make monosynaptic or fewer synaptic relays. As a result a more localized, specific and controllable response may be expected when they are activated as compared to C fibers.

Cutaneous receptor activation produces a high level of excitation to type II motor units and a high level of inhibition to type I motor units. Dynamic gamma motor neurons are also the most susceptible to cutaneous receptor activation. If these are not the motor units that are desired, therapeutic use of such stimulation will likely fail to provide the desired results and could perhaps produce adverse results.

Therapeutically, cutaneous input can be utilized for two general purposes:

1. Desensitization and inhibition: application of stimuli should be slow, firm maintained. Vibration is excellent for desensitizing the skin. It must be applied to the skin over a broad area. The vibrator should not be pushed into the muscle.

2. Facilitation of movement: application of stimuli should be quick, light and brief.

SECTION V

Summary of Patient Applications

CLINICAL APPLICATION SUMMARY

1. You have a "typical" patient you wish to treat. The patient has had a CVA and has spastic hemiparesis. What is your approach?

   It is difficult, most likely impossible, to make generalizations as to the practical application of the foregoing neurophysiology to a specific patient or group of patients.

   A fundamental problem with the practice of physical therapy is that we sometimes attempt to make such generalizations. Even though it is clear that each patient is an individual we are prone, for example, to treat all those with spasticity in the same general way.

   In the preceeding pages we have described just how varied patients can be. Two patients with spasticity will not respond to the same treatment. Two children who present with hypoextensibility of the muscles inserting into the achilles tendon may have entirely different pathologic mechanisms which cause the problem. As you might expect, the treatments should most likely be different.

   One of our greatest needs in physical therapy is to perfect more useful ways to categorize patients with particular neuropathology so the most appropriate _____ is applied.

treatment

---

2. Various evaluation systems based on research findings may be of some help in obtaining objective data from patients with central nervous system disorders. Some of these are summarized here:
   1. the extent to which the patient can voluntarily suppress the tonic vibration reflex.
   2. the slope of the patient's response to rapid stretch.
   3. the use of EMG to obtain an objective recording of the patient's responses during movement and postural activities.

   A most useful approach is careful observation of the patient's response and ability to perform in various _____.

activities

3. Research by Sahrmann (1982) has shown that a hemiplegic patient who had no ability to isolate a contraction of the quadriceps muscles (as in a muscle test position) could activate them sufficiently when in a weight bearing position to produce an acceptable gait pattern.

Another patient who had isolated control of these muscles while sitting could not activate them in a weight-bearing pattern.

In this case the patient who appears to be the most deficient or handicapped in fact proved to be the most functional.

This evidence shows that findings in a nonweight-bearing activity may not be generalized to an activity which is done while the individual is _____ _____.

bearing weight

Movement must be evaluated in the context of the activity that is undertaken. Do not expect the same results in a different situation. If you train a patient to use vision, for example, what will happen in the dark?

If you want the patient to perform under certain conditions then you should train the patient under those _____.

conditions

---

4. No one has been able to document a reliable correlation between muscle testing grades and functional abilities. This is true even in patients with lower motor neuron disturbances or other such weaknesses (Rothstein, 1983). Evaluation for spinal cord levels and other types of diagnostic information can be gleaned from manual muscle testing. Functional correlations, however, have not been shown to exist.

One of the major reasons that such a correlation has not been forthcoming is most likely because muscle test positions and conditions do not relate to the conditions under which the muscle must perform in a _____ activity.

functional

5. Rothstein (1983) proposed the following questions as a route for obtaining the detailed description of muscular performance:
   1. can the patient generate enough tension
      a. can it be generated fast enough
      b. is there a lack of tension at a specific point in the range
      c. can the patient generate the appropriate contractile mode (eccentric, isometric, isotonic, etc.)
   2. is there an inability to generate tension repeatedly
   3. can the muscle respond to training

   These statements show us that all muscle "weakness" is not the _____.

same

---

6. A patient working in a non-weight bearing activity may not produce any relevant results which can be carried over to a _____ _____ activity.

weight bearing

---

7. Working with concentric contractions may not produce the control needed during _____ contractions.

eccentric

---

8. Patients with upper motor neuron lesions manifest many different types of control problems. We have discussed the deficits in timing, sequence of muscle activity, the ability to generate tension quickly and to release it rapidly.

   Too often we have assumed all of these patients have the same deficits and have treated them accordingly.

   Appropriate therapeutic intervention requires that the patient's responses to the treatment be carefully _____.

monitored,
observed
or
categorized

9. If timing and sequencing of muscle activity are problems then therapeutic intervention should include activities which try to restore or develop the correct pattern of activation.

It has been very easy to assume that a patient who falls off the tilt board has a defective equilibrium response. It has been shown, however, that some such patients have an inappropriate sequence of activation of muscle groups (Horak, 1984). Yet, we may tend to treat all such patients with activities by manipulating the vestibular system.

It is important that treatment be based on clear and precise observations and not on _____.

assumptions

Much of the difficulty in communicating the results of patient evaluation and treatment is related to the use of terms which do not have the same meaning for all practitioners. Rather than suggest a patient has "increased tone" it may be more appropriate to describe the patient's motor behavior under various conditions utilizing universally accepted _____.

terminology

---

10. As therapists we are concerned with the fact that the patient does not have normal smooth coordinated movement. The difficulty lies in attempting to manipulate the defective or apparently defective motor output of patients with upper motor neuron lesions.

There is little that can be done to alter the motor output directly. The motor neurons are not spontaneously active and require input from the periphery and from descending tracts to activate them.

Armed with this information, therapists have devised numerous techniques for the application of peripheral sensory stimuli.

It is possible to change the motor behavior by manipulating the _____ input.

sensory

11. In the following discussion we will summarize various possible avenues for the manipulation of peripheral input. Please keep in mind that there is no "cook book" to give you. Careful observation of the stimulus and response should help direct you as to the appropriateness of any therapeutic intervention.

In order to effectively manipulate the motor output it is necessary to understand the characteristics of the neuromuscular components we wish to manipulate.

If motor neurons and muscle fibers consist of subgroups which are functionally organized, then knowledge of these components will assist us in prescribing or evaluating _____.

treatment

---

12. We have classified motor units into three basic types. There are many qualities and characteristics which are unique to each type of motor unit.

An understanding of these characteristics and how the units function will aid us in developing _____ strategies.

treatment

---

13. Type I motor units have the lowest threshold of activation and are capable of sustaining contraction for an extended period of time. We know that generally these motor units are recruited first and produce sustained activity.

It is very easy to hypothesize that these units work only in postural activities and provide the "proximal stability" which seems most desirable.

There are two possible problems with our hypothesis:
1. at least some of these motor units are recruited in all movements.
2. proximal stability may not always be what it appears to be, or what we have assumed it to be.

The muscles which initiate the most stable postural response may not be proximal muscles, but rather may be _____ muscles.

distal

347

14. Movements cannot be simplified into a scenario in which a contraction follows sensory input. Many factors have to be considered. For instance, does the specific sensory input being utilized have a greater influence on type II motor units than type I? Is that the type of motor unit which was desired?

The conditions under which a type of motor unit can be recruited preferentially are probably limited. Nonetheless, appropriate activity may enhance the probability of activation of specific motor units.

A marathon runner may have a predominance of type I fibers, but in order to capitalize on this endowment he or she must also run as an exercise activity to prepare for competition. Weight lifting or javalin throwing will not adequately prepare this athlete for long distance running.

The specific nature of the exercise will enhance the specific characteristics of the required _____ units.

motor

---

15. An individual with a greater proportion of type II motor units in a particular muscle group may fatigue more rapidly in an endurance activity and fail to protect the joints adequately.

This activity could result in joint or soft tissue _____ (Rose & Rothstein, 1983).

injury

---

16. An individual with a predominance of type I motor units may suffer joint and soft tissue injury because of an inability to generate sufficient tension rapidly if a sudden _____ is encountered (Rose & Rothstein, 1983).

load

---

17. Patients naturally have different motor unit proportions in their muscles. Additional complications arise because many diseases alter these proportions by specifically producing pathological changes in particular types of _____ _____.

motor units

18. The ability of the patient to produce sustained contractions or react to a sudden load may be significantly different than it was prior to his disease or injury because there has been a change in his muscle fiber type _____ .

predominance
or
proportion

---

19. It is impossible, therefore, to expect the same exercise or facilitation technique to produce the same response on a particular individual before and after his injury or illness.

Likewise, do not expect the same facilitation technique to produce the same response with _____ patients.

different

---

20. It has been demonstrated that muscles may have different characteristics depending upon their location in the body.

Tokizane and Shimazu (1964) have shown that tonic motor units in the lower extremity tend to have stronger tonic characteristics than do those same type of units in the upper extremity. Therefore, variation in response to treatment could be expected when comparing the upper and lower extremities.

We can determine whether an appropriate response is obtained through careful and continuous _____ .

observation

---

21. If you wish to activate the most tonic muscles or portions of muscles, the most likely candidates are the more medial and _____ muscles.

deeper

---

22. There is a greater projection from the primary afferent receptors onto the type _____ motor units.

I

muscle spindle

23. Stimuli which are most likely to activate the small slow to fatigue types of motor units are stretch, contraction, or vibration as these stimuli activate the _____ _____.

---

stretch

24. Sustained contractions continue the muscle spindle output to the alpha motor neurons through fusimotor system activation.

Slow contractions, especially against resistance, will be augmented by reflex support from the _____ reflex.

---

lower extremity

25. Stretch reflexes are particularly well developed in the anti-gravity muscles. So the anti-gravity muscles are the most suited to activation by this stimulus.

In addition, the anti-gravity muscles of the lower extremity are more tonic than those of the upper extremity.

It would appear likely that the muscles which will respond best to stretch reflex augmentation are those anti-gravity muscles of the _____ _____.

---

reciprocal inhibition

26. Strong sustained activation of the desired muscles should produce inhibition of the antagonists through the phenomenon of _____ _____.

---

antagonists

27. If specific inhibition to a muscle group is desired, it may be accomplished, therefore, by activation of the _____.

28. A strong contraction of the agonist may also be followed by inhibition or relaxation of that muscle.

This may happen because of strong activation of the _____.

GTO's
(and some joint receptors,
particularly type III)

---

29. There may be secondary receptors in muscles which are specifically excitatory to flexors. The secondary receptors are most strongly activated near the end of the range of motion.

The GTO's are also most strongly activated under certain circumstances when the muscle is most fully elongated. The GTO's produce a stronger effect in extensor muscles.

If your goal is to activate extensor muscles then it may be useful to work with the extensor muscle in the area of the joint range of motion we have called the _____ _____.

submaximum range

---

30. According to Wyke (1979) type I joint receptors project generally to the type I motor units.

Again, if your goal is to attempt stronger activation of the type I motor units, utilization of joint input designed to activate type I receptors would seem reasonable.

The stimulus necessary to activate the type I receptors is sustained movement or pressure involving the _____ joints.

proximal

---

31. In general, the reflex circuits in which joint receptors participate tend to provide excitation primarily to the _____ muscles.

extensor

32. If you wish to test the arthrokinetic and arthrostatic reflexes, the former is best accomplished by examining the proximal joints.

The latter requires a set up to evaluate postural responses while the individual is in a _____ _____ position.

weight bearing

---

33. Balance boards and rocking chairs provide some avenues for treatment of impaired kinesthetic sense and _____ and _____ reflexes.

kinesthetic
arthrostatic

---

34. Some of the cutaneous fibers which are supplied by the larger axons may facilitate type I motor units.

The modality that you might use which is most likely to accomplish type I facilitation is firm _____ or _____.

touch
pressure

---

35. The large motor units are highly cortically driven, are very fatiguable, and are movement oriented. These fibers are less "postural" in the sense that they do not sustain contractions over a long period. They are the fibers which generate the greatest tension.

We have already indicated that some type II motor units will participate in both tonic and phasic activities. Certainly not all type II motor units will be involved in the more tonic activities.

It is clear that some motor units are best suited for steady sustained contractions at particular levels of activity. When considering the combined pool of motor neurons it is likely that some are better recruited in one type of activity than another.

If you wish to emphasize the activation of type I motor units it is likely the following stimuli would be most effective: _____
_____
_____

movement, voluntary activity, reciprocal movement of distal joints (type II joint receptors) most types of cutaneous input

extensors

36. Cutaneous input tends to produce a net effect of facilitation of the flexor muscles and inhibition of the _____.

---

37. Information concerning synaptic patterns involving type I and type II motor units leads us to certain precautions.

When considering the role of proprioceptive and exteroceptive input during exercise it appears that some input may make it easier to recruit one type of motor unit than another.

We will have to wonder whether stimulation-induced contraction will actually produce a "normal" contraction (Rothstein, 1983).

Extrapolation of neurophysiologic research to the clinical setting requires caution. It is critical that the therapist carefully and continually monitor the patient's _____ to treatment.

response

---

38. Co-contraction or co-activation of the agonists and antagonists has been identified by some therapists as a necessary ingredient in some treatment procedures because some patients appear to lack co-contraction and demonstrate instability.

There are some points we should remember on this subject, and the first one is that recent studies have shown us that often the most stable patient is not the one in whom the agonists and antagonists are co-activated during certain activities (Horak, 1984).

If co-contraction is desirable it appears to be possible to produce it through activation of the extensors.If the extensor is undergoing contraction in the maximum range both the secondary receptors which may be specifically excitatory to flexors and the GTO will be the most stimulated.

The net result will be activation of the flexors through certain of the secondary receptors and the GTO, and activation of the extensors through the _____ receptor.

primary

39. It should be appropriate here to consider the responses of the secondary receptors as they relate to the problems of patient treatment.

The classical concept of the function of the secondary receptor as being excitatory to flexors and inhibitory to extensors has been found to hold true in at least certain muscles in man in the presence of spinal cord injury. This finding is in agreement with the findings in spinal cats (Burke, et.al., 1970, 1971).

Studies of patients with injuries higher in the central nervous system do not show the same responses. It is apparent that the secondary receptors can participate in a variety of reflex actions depending upon the integrity and state of the CNS (Urbscheit, 1979).

Patient populations have not yet been classified as to the particular response which may be expected from a patient with a certain type of pathological condition.

The variation of reflex responses mediated by this secondary receptor serve to show us that there is yet much we do not know about the nervous system and its functions. This variability also points out the danger in dogmatic acceptance or adherence to particular techniques which may be utilized in patient treatment.

One should not expect that the reflex response will be the same in all patients nor that the same treatment approach will be beneficial to all patients. It is clear that neither simple nor complex reflex responses should constitute the sole basis for patient _____.

treatment

---

40. Investigators have shown that reflexes which are mediated or supported by the secondary receptors are not identical in all circumstances.

Secondary receptors can participate in a variety of reflex actions depending upon the integrity and state of the _____.

CNS

41. A newer understanding of the probable mechanisms in spasticity should be most helpful in patient treatment.

If the deficit in spasticity involves the central gaining mechanism rather than excessive driving of the fusimotor neurons and muscle spindles which are overly sensitive it is clear that the older view of "biasing the spindles to new lengths" is invalid.

Many of the specific techniques utilized to control spasticity are still quite useful. That is stretch, vibration, resisted contraction, touch, pressure and so forth may still be utilized to facilitate a desired response.

It is helpful to understand that our reasons for using these techniques may change because research continues to clarify and add to our knowledge of these things. Most of these techniques were developed because they appeared at least empirically to work in the clinical setting.

It stands to reason that techniques were first developed as a result of good clinical observation they may still be utilized in the presence of good clinical _____.

observation

---

42. It is important to remember that all receptors have projections to higher centers. Most if not all types of sensory information is relayed to the cortex for conscious awareness.

Sending information to these centers is among the most important reasons for using sensory input in patient treatment. Such feedback appears to be useful in motor learning tasks, and in giving an individual a "feel" for the correct movement or response.

You may help him to do so by providing _____ _____.

sensory input

43. We maintain that very little damage will be done to a patient if an incorrect facilitation or inhibition technique is utilized briefly to ascertain the appropriateness of the response it elicits.

The damage which is done to patients occurs when the therapist continues the treatment program and repeats the same conditions and elicits the same responses when they are in fact not desirable.

If a person can walk on an ankle that has no range of motion does it make sense to increase that range of motion? What if there is no voluntary control of the muscles acting over that joint? Increasing the range of motion, in this case, will prove disabling to the patient. With a larger range of motion and no control over this joint the patient will now have to be braced for stability.

Anyone who is trying to achieve more range of motion should test the patient to find out if any voluntary activity exists but is masked by the contracture. If not, range of motion treatments should cease immediately.

Good patient care involves thinking through the problem and making careful observations of the _____ _____.

treatment results

___

44. Peripheral input or the suppression of peripheral input may assist your treatment but it should rarely if ever be the sole avenue of treatment. Recognition that timing, sequencing, generation of adequate tension and appropriate release of tension as the most important components of movement tells us that peripheral control of movement is not only limited but in some instances inappropriate.

Knowledge concerning Higher levels of motor control must be coordinated with information about peripheral influences on _____ _____.

motor control

45. It is extremely important to understand that structural and functional changes which occur secondary to CNS lesions are ongoing from seconds to years.

If the changes are occuring 24 hours a day treatment may have to span 24 hours a day. The most critical part of the therapists program may be training other professional support personnel and the patient's family and friends, as well as the patient, to maintain treatment when the therapist is not present.

Treatment which is given 24 hours a day may prevent or alter the structural and functional changes which contribute to spasticity, and therefore, control the development of _____.

spasticity

---

46. With alterations in patterns of activity there are likely to be alterations in musculoskeletal balance. If short, tight muscles are present (antagonists lengthened) the resulting mechanical imbalance may produce pain. Painful inputs will further alter function.

One of the fundamental considerations in treatment must be to correct posture and musculo-skeletal _____ (Kendall & McCreary, 1983; Sahrmann, 1983).

imbalances

---

47. With disorders of muscle tone, it takes time to fully develop all the morphological changes that may occur in spasticity and cause permanent changes.

These observations tell us that **early** treatment is of the essence for optimal results.

Early treatment may prevent the development of lasting _____ responses.

abnormal

48. We are obliged to consider the patient's condition 24 hours a day. Other personnel and family may have to be educated and the environment may have to be _____.

modified

Peripheral input can assist or detract from central mechanisms. Choose wisely, apply carefully, observe diligently.

Selecting the appropriate treatment for each patient depends upon numerous conditions. Researchers have made some progress in defining certain conditions. For example, EMG studies of elbow flexors during passive elbow flexion and extension show some expected and some unexpected results. A lengthening or stretch response in the elbow flexors would be expected when the muscles are lengthened or stretched as the elbow joint is extended. It was also noted that normal individuals have a "shortening response". This response is an EMG burst when the joint is passively moved into the shortened range (Sahrmann & Norton, 1977).

Sahrmann has shown that the shortening response of spastic patients is not as strong as in normals. In some patients they are absent. Follow-up studies have shown that those patients with a shortening response have a better recovery than those who do not show this response.

Such studies indicate that our ability to categorize patients according to predictable criteria would greatly enhance our knowledge of how to treat certain patients and how to predict treatment outcomes.

Obviously, **research** is needed in every facet of physical therapy.

BIBLIOGRAPHY

BIBLIOGRAPHY

Anderson, P., and J. Henriksson: Training-induced changes in the subgroups of human type II skeletal muscle fibers. Acta Physiol Scand, 99: 392-397, 1977.

Andrews, C.J., D. Burke and J.W. Lance: The response to muscle stretch and shortening in Parkinsonian rigidity. Brain, 95: 795-812, 1972.

Andrews, C.J., P.D. Neilson and L. Knowles: Electromyographic study of the rigido-spasticity of athetosis. J Neurol Neurosurg Psychiat, 36: 94-103, 1973a.

Andrews, C.J., P.D. Neilson and J.W. Lance: Comparison of stretch reflexes and shortening reactions in activated normal subjects with those in Parkinson's Disease. J Neurol Neurosurg Psychiat, 36: 329-333, 1973b.

Appelberg, B., M. Hulliger and H. Johansson: Excitation of dynamic fusimotor neurons of the cat triceps surae by contralateral joint afferents. Brain Res, 160: 529-532, 1979.

Ashby, P. and D. Burke: Stretch reflexes in the upper limb of spastic man. J Neurol Neurosurg Psychiat, 34: 765-771, 1971.

Baldissera, F., H. Hultborn and M. Illert: Integration in spinal neuronal systems. In J.M. Brookhart and V.B. Mountcastle, Eds: Handbook of Physiology, Section 1: The Nervous System, American Physiological Society, Bethesda, MD., 1981.

Barker, D.: The innervation of mammalian skeletal muscle. In A.V. De Reuck and J. Knight, Eds., Myotatic, Kinesthetic and Vestibular Mechanisms, Ciba, 1967.

Basmajian, J.V.: Muscles Alive, 3rd Ed., Williams and Wilkins, 1978.

Bishop, B.: Spasticity: its physiology and management. Monograph Amer Phys Ther Assn, 1977.

Bishop, B.: Basic Neurophysiology, Medical Examination Publishing Co., New York, 1982.

Bishop, B. and R.L. Craik: Neural Plasticity. Monograph Amer Phys Ther Assn, 1982.

Boyd, I.A.: The mechanical properties of dynamic nuclear bag fibers, static nuclear bag fibers and nuclear chain fibers in isolated cat muscle spindles. Prog Brain Res, 44: 33-66, 1976.

Brooke, M.H. and K.K. Kaiser: Muscle fiber types: how many and what kind?, Arch Neurol 23: 369-379, 1970.

Brooke, M.H., E. Williamson and K.K. Kaiser: The behavior of four fiber types in developing reinnervated muscle. Arch Neurol, 25: 360-366, 1971.

Bryan, R.N., et.al.: Evidence for a common location of alpha and gamma motoneurons. Brain Res, 38: 193-196, 1972.

Buller, A.J., J.C. Eccles and R.M. Eccles: Interactions between motoneurons and muscles in respect of the characteristic speeds of their responses. J Physiol, 150: 417-439, 1960.

Burke, D., J.D. Gillies and J.W. Lance: The quadriceps stretch reflex in human spasticity. J Neurol Neurosurg Psychiat, 33: 216-223, 1970.

Burke, D., J.D. Gillies and J.W. Lance: Hamstring stretch reflex in human spasticity. J Neurol Neurosurg Psychiat, 34: 321-325, 1971.

Burke, D., K. Hagbarth and L. Lofstedt: Muscle spindle activity in man during shortening and lengthening contractions. J Physiol, 277: 131-142, 1978.

Burke, D.: The activity of human muscle spindle endings in normal motor behavior. In Porter, R., Ed. International Review of Physiology, Neurophysiology IV, University Park Press, Baltimore, MD., 1980.

Burke, D.: Critical examination of the case for or against fusimotor involvement in disorders of muscle tone. In J.E. Desmedt, Ed., Motor Control Mechanisms in Health and Disease, Raven Press, New York, 1983.

Burke, R.E.: Motor unit types of cat triceps surae muscle. J Physiol, 193: 141-160, 1967.

Burke, R.E., D.N. Levine, F.E. Zajac, and P. Tsairis: Mammalian motor units, physiological-histochemical correlation in three types of motor units in cat gastrocnemius. Science, 174: 709-712, 1971.

Burke, R.E.: On the central nervous system control of fast and slow twitch motor units. In New Developments in Electromyography and Clinical Neurophysiology. Vol 3, Karger, Switzerland, 1973.

Burke, R.E.: Motor units in mammalian muscle. In Summer A. Ed., The physiology of peripheral nerve disease, W.B. Saunders, Philadelphia, 1980.

Burke, R.E.: Motor units: anatomy, physiology, and functional organization. In J.M. Brookhart and V.B. Mountcastle, Eds: Handbook of Physiology, Section 1: The Nervous System, American Physiological Society, Bethesda, MD., 1981.

Castle, M.E., T.A. Reyman and M. Schneider: Pathology of spastic muscle in cerebral palsy. Clin Ortho Rel Res, Lippincott, 1979.

Crago, P.E., J.C. Houk and Z. Hasan: Regulatory actions of the human stretch reflex. J Neurophysiol, 39: 925-935, 1976.

Cummings, G.: Personal Communication, 1984.

Duchenne, G.B.: Physiology of motion. J.B. Lippincott, Philadelphia, 1949.

Edgerton, V.R.: Neuromuscular adaptation to power and endurance work. Canadian J Appl Sport Sci, 1: 49-58, 1976.

Eldred, E., H. Schnitzlein, and J. Buchwald: Response of muscle spindles to stimulation of sympathetic trunks. Exp Neurol, 13-24, 1960.

Evarts, E.: Motor cortex reflexes associated with learned movement. Science, 179: 501-503, 1973.

Granit, R.: The basis of motor control. Academic Press, New York, 1970.

Hagbarth, K.E.: Excitatory and inhibitory skin areas for flexor and extensor motoneurons. Acta Physiol Scand, 26 (Suppl 94), Stockholm, 1952.

Hagbarth, K.E. and G. Eklund: The effects of muscle vibration in spasticity, rigidity, and cerebellar disorders. J Neurol Neurosurg Psych, 31: 207-213, 1968.

Hagbarth, K.E. and G. Eklund: Tonic vibration reflexes in spasticity. Brain Res, 2: 201-203, 1966.

Harris, D. and E. Henneman: Different species of alpha motoneurons in the same pool: further evidence from the effects of inhibition in their firing rates. J Neurophysiol, 42, 1979.

Henneman, E.: Organization of the motor neuron pool: the size principle. In V.B. Mountcastle, Ed., Med Physiol, 14th ed., C.V. Mosby, St. Louis, MO., 1980.

Henneman, E. and L. Mendell: Functional organization of the motoneuron pool and its inputs. In J.M. Brookhart and V.B. Mountcastle, Eds. Handbook of Physiology, Section 1: The Nervous System, American Physiological Society, Bethesda, MD., 1981.

Homma, S., K. Ishikawa and S. Watanabe: Optimal frequency of muscle vibration for motor neuron firing. J China Med Soc, 43: 190-196, 1967.

Hong, K., W. Janig and R. Schmidt: Properties of group IV fibers in the nerves to the knee joint of the cat. J Physiol (London), 284: 178-179, 1978.

Horak, F.B.: Disorders of Posture and Movement: Control Variables. Presented at 1984 American Physical Therapy Association Mid-Winter Conference.

Houk, J.C. and W.Z. Rymer: Neural control of muscle length and tension. In J.M. Brookhart and V.B. Mountcastle, Eds., Handbook of Physiology, Section 1: The Nervous System, American Physiological Society, Bethesda, MD., 1981.

Hutter, O.F. and W.R. Loewenstein: Nature of neuromuscular facilitation by sympathetic stimulation in the frog. J Physiol, 130: 559, 1955.

Jaweed, M.M., G.J. Herbison and J.F. Ditunno: Myosin ATPase activity after strengthening exercise. J Anat, 124: 371-381, 1977.

Johnson, R.M., B. Bishop and G.H. Coffey: Mechanical vibration of skeletal muscles. Phys Ther, 50(4): 499-505, 1970.

Johnstone, M.: Restoration of motor function in the stroke patient. Churchill Livingstone, New York, 1983.

Kandel, E.R. and J.H. Schwartz: Principles of Neural Science, Elsevier, New York, 1981.

Kendall, F.P. and E.K. McCreary: Muscles testing and function. Williams and Wilkins, Baltimore, MD., 1983.

Lance, J.W., D.J. Burke, P.D. Neilson and D.G. Milder: A physiological approach to motor disorders. Contemp Clin Neurophys (EEG Suppl No 34), W.A. Cobb and H. Van Duijn, Eds., Elsevier Co., Amsterdam, 1978.

Lundberg, A.: Control of spinal mechanisms from the brain. In D.B. Tower, Ed. The Nervous System, Vol 1, The Basic Neurosciences, New York, Raven Press, 1975.

McCafferty, W.V., and S.M. Horvath: Specificity of exercise and specificity of training: a subcellular review. Res Quart Am Assoc Health Phy Educ, 48 (2): 358-371, 1977.

Marsden, C.D.: Servo control, the stretch reflex and movement in man. In Desmedt, J.E., Ed.: Progress in Clinical Neurophysiology, Vol 4. Karger, Switzerland, 1978.

Maton, B.: Fast and slow motor units: their recruitment for tonic and phasic contraction in normal man. Eur J Appl Physiol, 43: 45-55, 1980.

Matthews, P.: Evidence that the secondary as well as the primary endings of the muscle spindles may be responsible for the tonic stretch reflex of the decrebrate cat. J Physiol, 204: 365-393, 1969.

Melzack, R. and P.D. Wall: Pain mechanisms: a new theory. Science, 150: 971-979, 1965.

Mendell, L.M. and E. Henneman: Terminals of single Ia fibers: location and density and distribution within a pool of 300 homonymous motoneurons. J Neurophysiol, 34: 171-187, 1971.

Mountcastle, V.B. Ed.: Medical Physiology, 14th Edition, C.V. Mosby, St. Louis, MO., 1980.

Munsat, T.L., McNeal D., Waters, R.: Effects of nerve stimulation on human muscle. Arch Neurol, 33: 608, 1976.

Nathan, P.: Some comments on spasticity and rigidity. In Desmedt, J.E., Ed., New Developments in Electromyography and Clinical Neurophysiology, Karger, Switzerland, 1973.

Neilson, P.D.: Voluntary and reflex control of the biceps brachii muscle in spastic-athetotic patients. J Neurol Neurosurg Psychiat, 35: 853-860, 1972a.

Neilson, P.D.: Interaction between voluntary contraction and tonic stretch reflex transmission in normal and spastic patients. J Neurol Neurosurg Psychiat, 35: 589-598, 1972b.

Nelson, S.G. and E. Mendell: Projection of single semitendinosus Ia afferent fibers to homonymous and heteronymous motoneurons. J Physiol, 41: 778, 1978.

Newton, R.: Joint receptor contributions to reflexive and kinesthetic responses. Phys Ther, 62: 22-29, 1982.

Odeen, I. and E. Knutsson: Evaluation of the effects of muscle stretch and weight load in patients with spastic paraplegia. Scand J Rehab Med, 13: 117-121, 1981.

O'Connell, A.L. and E.B. Gardner: Ingredients of coordinate movement. Am J Phys Med, 46: 334-361, 1967.

Pansky, B. and D.J. Allen: Review of Neuroscience. Macmillan, New York, 1980.

Patten, B.M.: Human Embryology, McGraw-Hill, New York, 1953.

Patton, N.J. and O. Mortenson: An electromyographic study of reciprocal activity of muscles. Anatom Rec, 170: 255-268, 1971.

Peter, J.B., J. Barnard, V.R. Edgerton, C.A. Gillespie and K.E. Stemple: Metabolic profiles of three fiber types of skeletal muscle in guinea pigs and rabbits. Biochemistry, 11: 2627-2633, 1972.

Pette, D., Muller, W., Leisner, E., and Vrbova, G.: Time-dependent effects on contractile properties, fiber population, myosin light chains, and enzymes of energy metabolism in intermittent and continuously stimulated fast-twitch muscle of the rabbit. Pfluegers Archiv, 364: 103-112, 1976.

Pette, D., Ed.: Plasticity of Muscle. Gruyter, Berlin, 1980.

Rose, S.J. and J.M. Rothstein: Muscle Mutability: Part 1. General concepts and adaptations to altered pattern of use. Muscle Biology, Monograph Amer Phys Ther Assn, 1983.

Rothstein, J.M.: Muscle Biology: Clinical Considerations. Muscle Biology, Monograph Amer Phys Ther Assn, 1983.

Sahrmann, S.A. and B.J. Norton: The relationship of voluntary movement to spasticity in the upper motor neuron syndrome. Anals of Neurology, 2: 460-465, 1977.

Sahrmann, S.A. and B.J. Norton: Stretch reflex of the biceps and brachioradialis muscles in patients with upper motor neuron syndrome. Phys Ther, 58: 1191-1194, 1978.

Sahrmann, S.A.: A program for correction of muscular imbalance and mechanical imbalance. Clinical Management, 3: 23-28, 1983.

Saito, M., M. Tomonaga and K. Hirayama: Histochemical study of normal human muscle spindle: histochemical classification of intrafusal muscle fibers and intrafusal nerve endings. J Neurol, 216: 79-89, 1977.

Scholz, J.P. and S.K. Campbell: Muscle spindles and the regulation of movement. Phys Ther, 60: 1416-1423, 1980.

Stacey, M.J.: Free nerve endings in skeletal muscle of the cat. J Anat, 105: 231-254, 1969.

Stockmeyer, S.A.: An interpretation of the approach of rood to the treatment of neuromuscular dysfunction. Am J Phys Med, 46: 900-956, 1967.

Stuart, D.G.: Conditional nature of spinal reflexes. Read at the Missouri APTA Fall Meeting, St. Louis, MO., 1981.

Swash, M. and K. Fox: Muscle spindle innervation in man. J Anat, 112: 61-80, 1972.

Tabary, J., C. Tardieu, G. Tardieu and C. Tabary: Experimental rapid sarcomere loss with concomitant hypoextensibility. Muscle and Nerve, 4: 198-203, 1981.

Tardieu, C., E. Heut de la Tour and G. Tardieu: Muscle hypoextensibility in children with cerebral palsy: I. clinical and experimental observations. Arch Phys Med Rehabil, March 1982.

Tardieu, G., C. Tardieu, P. Colbeau-Justin and A. Lespargot: Muscle hypoextensibility in children with cerebral palsy: II therapeutic implications. Arch Phys Med Rehabil, March 1982.

Tokizane, T. and H. Shimazu: Functional differentiation of human skeletal muscle-- corticalization and spinalization of movement. Charles Thomas, Springfield, IL., 1964.

Truscella, D., A. Lespargot, and G. Tardieu: Variation in the long-term results of elongation of the tendo achillis in children with cerebral palsy. J Bone Jt Surg, 61-B, No 4, 1979.

Urbscheit, N.L.: Reflexes evoked by group II afferent fibers from muscle spindles. Phys Ther, 59: 1083-1087, 1979.

Vallbo, A.B.: Muscle spindle response at the onset of isometric voluntary contractions in man. Time difference between fusimotor and skeletomotor effects. J Physiol (London), 218: 405-431, 1971.

Vander, A.J., J.H. Sherman and D.S. Luciano: Human physiology, the mechanisms of body function. McGraw-Hill, New York, 1980.

Vrbova, G.: Influence of activity on some characteristic properties of slow and fast mammilian muscles. J Physiol, 252: 181-213, 1979.

Wyke, B.: Articular neurology--a review. Chart Soc of Physiotherp, 94-99, 1972.

Wyke, B.: Articular neurology. Read at the National Conference of the APTA, Atlanta, GA., 1979.

INDEX